Histological Typing of Ovarian Tumours

Springer-Verlag Berlin Heidelberg GmbH

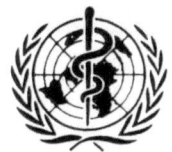 World Health Organization

The series *International Histological Classification of Tumours* consists of the following volumes. The early ones can be ordered through WHO, Distribution and Sales, Avenue Appia, CH-1211 Geneva 27.

  1. Histological typing of lung tumours (1967, second edition 1981)
  2. Histological typing of breast tumours (1968, second edition 1981)
10. Histological typing of urinary bladder tumours (1973)
14. Histological and cytological typing of neoplastic diseases of haematopoietic and lymphoid tissues (1976)
22. Histological typing of prostate tumours (1980)
23. Histological typing of endocrine tumours (1980)

A coded compendium of the International Histological Classification of Tumours (1978).

The following volumes have already appeared in a revised second edition with Springer-Verlag:
Histological Typing of Thyroid Tumours. Hedinger/Williams/Sobin (1988)
Histological Typing of Intestinal Tumours. Jass/Sobin (1989)
Histological Typing of Oesophageal and Gastric Tumours. Watanabe/Jass/Sobin (1990)
Histological Typing of Tumours of the Gallbladder and Extrahepatic Bile Ducts. Albores-Saavedra/Henson/Sobin (1990)
Histological Typing of Tumours of the Upper Respiratory Tract and Ear. Shanmugaratnam/Sobin (1981)
Histological Typing of Salivary Gland Tumours. Seifert (1991)
Histological Typing of Odontogenic Tumours. Kramer/Pindborg/Shear (1992)
Histological Typing of Tumours of the Central Nervous System. Kleihues/Burger/Scheithauer (1993)
Histological Typing of Bone Tumours. Schajowicz (1993)
Histological Typing of Soft Tissue Tumours. Weiss (1994)
Histological Typing of Female Genital Tract Tumours. Scully et al. (1994)
Histological Typing of Tumours of the Liver. Ishak et al. (1994)
Histological Typing of Tumours of the Exocrine Pancreas. Klöppel/Solcia/Longnecker/Capella/Sobin (1996)
Histological Typing of Skin Tumours. Heenan/Elder/Sobin (1996)
Histological Typing of Cancer and Precancer of the Oral Mucosa. Pindborg/Reichart/Smith/van der Waal (1997)
Histological Typing of Kidney Tumours. Mostofi/Davis (1998)
Histological Typing of Testis Tumours. Mostofi/Sesterhenn (1998)
Histological Typing of Tumours of the Eye and Its Adnexa. Campbell (1998)
Histological Typing of Ovarian Tumours. Scully (1999)

Histological Typing of Ovarian Tumours

R.E. Scully

In Collaboration with L.H. Sobin
and Pathologists in 5 Countries

Second Edition

With 130 Colour Figures, 20 Black and White Figures
and an Appendix on TNM Staging with 9 Black and White Figures

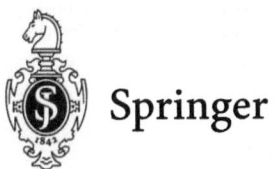 Springer

Robert E. Scully, MD
James Homer Wright Laboratories, Massachusetts General Hospital
32 Fruit Street, WRN 242, Boston, MA 02114-2696, USA

Leslie H. Sobin
WHO Collaborating Center for the International Histological
Classification of Tumours, Armed Forces Institute of Pathology
Washington, DC 20306-6000, USA

First edition published by WHO in 1980 as No. 9 in the International Histological
Classification of Tumours series

ISBN 978-3-540-64059-2

Library of Congress Cataloging-in-Publication Data
Scully, Robert E. (Robert Edward), 1921- Histological typing of ovarian tumours. - 2nd ed./R.E.
Scully, in collaboration with L.H. Sobin and pathologists in 5 countries. p. cm. - (Histological classi-
fication of tumours) Rev. ed. of: Histological typing of ovarian tumours/S.F. Serov, R.E. Scully, in col-
laboration with L.H. Sobin ... 1973. Includes bibliographical references and index.
ISBN 978-3-540-64059-2   ISBN 978-3-642-58564-7 (eBook)
DOI 10.1007/978-3-642-58564-7
1. Ovaries-Tumors-Histopathology. 2. Ovaries-Tumors-Classification. I. Sobin, L.H. II. Serov, S.F.
(Sergeĭ Fedorovich). Histological typing of ovarian tumours. III. Title. IV. Series.
[DNLM: 1. Ovarian Neoplasms-classification. 2. Ovarian Neoplasms-pathology.   WP 15   S437h
1999] RC280.08S38 1999 616.99'265-dc21 DNLM/DLC 99-10480

© Springer-Verlag Berlin Heidelberg 1999
Originally published by Springer-Verlag Berlin Heidelberg New York in 1999

The use of general descriptive names, registered names, trademarks, etc. in this publication does not
imply, even in the absence of a specific statement, that such names are exempt from the relevant pro-
tective laws and regulations and therefore free for general use.

Product liability: The publisher cannot guarantee the accuracy of any information about dosage and
application contained in this book. In every individual case the user must check such information by
consulting the relevant literature.

SPIN: 10765018   24/3111 – 5 4 3 2 1 – Printed on acid-free paper.

Participants

Fox, H., Dr.
Department of Pathological Sciences, University of Manchester,
Manchester, UK

Russell, P., Dr.
Department of Anatomical Pathology, University of Sidney,
Sydney, Australia

Saksela, E., Dr.
Department of Pathology, University of Helsinki,
Helsinki, Finland

Sasano, N., Dr.
Department of Pathology, Tohoku University School of Medicine,
Sendai, Japan

Scully, R.E., Dr.
James Homer Wright Laboratories, Massachusetts General Hospital,
Boston, MA, USA

Sobin, L.H., Dr.
WHO Collaborative Center for the International Histological
Classification of Tumours, Armed Forces Institute of Pathology,
Washington, DC, USA

Talerman, A., Dr.
Department of Pathology and Cell Biology,
Thomas Jefferson University, Philadelphia, PA, USA

General Preface to the Series

Among the prerequisites for comparative studies of cancer are international agreement on histological criteria for the definition and classification of cancer types and a standardized nomenclature. An internationally agreed classification of tumours, acceptable alike to physicians, surgeons, radiologists, pathologists and statisticians, would enable cancer workers in all parts of the world to compare their findings and would facilitate collaboration among them.

In a report published in 1952[1], a subcommittee of the World Health Organization (WHO) Expert Committee on Health Statistics discussed the general principles that should govern the statistical classification of tumours and agreed that, to ensure the necessary flexibility and ease of coding, three separate classifications were needed according to (1) anatomical site, (2) histological type, and (3) degree of malignancy. A classification according to anatomical site is available in the International Classification of Diseases[2].

In 1956, the WHO Executive Board passed a resolution[3] requesting the Director-General to explore the possibility that WHO might organize centres in various parts of the world and arrange for the collection of human tissues and their histological classification. The main purpose of such centres would be to develop histological definitions of cancer types and to facilitate the wide adoption of a uniform nomenclature. The resolution was endorsed by the Tenth World Health Assembly in May 1957[4].

Since 1958, WHO has established a number of centres concerned with this subject. The result of this endeavor has been the

---

[1] WHO (1952) WHO Technical Report Series, no. 53. WHO, Geneva, p. 45.

[2] WHO (1977) Manual of the international statistical classification of diseases, injuries, and causes of death, 1975 version. WHO, Geneva.

[3] WHO (1956) WHO Official Records, no. 68, p 14 (resolution EB 17.R40).

[4] WHO (1957) WHO Official Records, no. 79, p. 467 (resolution WHA 10.18).

International Histological Classification of Tumours, a multivolumed series whose first edition was published between 1967 and 1981. The present revised second edition aims to update the classifications, reflecting progress in diagnosis and the relevance of tumour types to clinical and epidemiological features.

Preface to Histological Typing of Ovarian Tumours - Second Edition

The first edition of *Histological Typing of Ovarian Tumours* was the result of the collaborative effort organized by WHO and carried out by the Collaborating Center for the Histological Classification of Ovarian Tumours at the Petrov Institute of Oncology Research in Leningrad, Soviet Union. The classification was published in 1973[1].

The task of updating the classification was given to the Classification and Nomenclature Committee of the International Society of Gynecological Pathologists. Classification proposals were discussed during meetings of the ovarian tumour subcommittee and presented orally to the members of the society during their general meeting. The classification was finally circulated to the society members for their suggestions, which were considered and discussed at the final meeting of the subcommittee.

The final classification reflects the present state of knowledge, and modifications will probably be needed as experience accumulates. It is therefore expected that some pathologists may dissent from certain aspects of the classification or terminology adopted in this volume. It is nevertheless hoped that in the interests of international cooperation and comparability of data, all pathologists will use the classification as put forward. Criticisms and suggestions for its improvement will be welcomed; these should be sent to the World Health Organization, Geneva, Switzerland.

The histological classification, which appears on pp. 3-9 contains the morphology code numbers of the *International Classification of*

---

[1] Serov SS, Scully RE, Sobin LH (1973) Histological typing of ovarian tumours Geneva, World Health Organization (International Histological Classification of Tumours, No. 9).

Diseases for Oncology (ICD-O)[2] and the *Systematized Nomenclature of Medicine* (SNOMED)[3].

The publications in the series, *International Histological Classification of Tumours* are not intended to serve as textbooks, butrather to promote the adoption of a uniform terminology that willfacilitate communication among cancer workers. For this reason,literature references have intentionally been omitted and readers should refer to standard works for bibliographies.

---

[2] World Health Geganization (1990) International classification of diseases for oncology (ICD-O),Geneva.
[3] College of American Pathologists (1982) Systematized nomenclature of medicine (SNOMED). Chicago, IL.

Contents

Introduction

Although the histological typing of ovarian tumours is the focus of this volume, other aspects of investigation of a specimen of ovarian tumour are also important. Some of these aspects are mentioned in the text or illustrated. They include tumour grading, which is important prognostically and therapeutically for certain types of ovarian tumour, quantification of components in mixed tumours and evaluation of the stroma of certain tumours that are associated with endocrine function. Grading methodologies have varied from one tumour type to another and from one group of investigators to another for the same type of tumour. Because a standard internationally recognized grading methodology has not been established, no specific guidance is presented in this volume. Nevertheless, grading by any generally acceptable method should be incorporated in the diagnosis whenever appropriate.

The clinical and pathological classification of the extent of tumour growth (staging) should be taken into account for the purposes of treatment and prognosis. The TNM/FIGO system is therefore included (p. 45).

Histological Classification of Ovarian Tumours

1   **Surface Epithelial-Stromal Tumours**

1.1	*Serous tumours*	
1.1.1	Benign	
1.1.1.1	Cystadenoma	8441/0[1]
	Papillary cystadenoma	8460/0
1.1.1.2	Surface papilloma	8461/0
1.1.1.3	Adenofibroma; cystadenofibroma	9014/0
1.1.2	Of borderline malignancy (of low malignant potential)	
1.1.2.1	*Cystic tumour*	*8442/1*[2]
	Papillary cystic tumour	*8462/1*
1.1.2.2	*Surface papillary tumour*	*8463/1*
1.1.2.3	Adenofibroma; cystadenofibroma	9014/1
1.1.3	Malignant	
1.1.3.1	Adenocarcinoma	8441/3
	Papillary adenocarcinoma	8460/3
	Papillary cystadenocarcinoma	8460/3
1.1.3.2	Surface papillary adenocarcinoma	8461/3
1.1.3.3	Adenocarcinofibroma; cystadenocarcinofibroma (malignant adenofibroma; cystadenofibroma) . . .	9014/3

---

[1] Morphology code of the International Classification of Disease for Oncology (ICD-O) and the Systematized Nomenclature of Medicine (SNOMED). Behaviour is coded /0 for benign tumours, /1 for low or uncertain malignant potential or borderlin malignancy, and /3 for malignant tumours.

[2] The italicized numbers are provisional codes proposed for the third edition of ICD-O. They should, for the most part, be incorporated into the next edition of ICD-O, but they are subject to change.

3   Germ Cell Tumours

5   Germ Cell – Sex Cord-Stromal Tumour of Non-gonadoblastoma Type

5.1   Variant – with dysgerminoma or other germ cell tumour

6   Tumours of Rete Ovarii

6.1   Adenoma 8140/0
        Cystadenoma 8440/0
6.2   Adenocarcinoma 8140/3

7   Mesothelial Tumours

7.1   Adenomatoid tumour 9054/0
7.2   Mesothelioma 9050/3

8   Tumours of Uncertain Origin and Miscellanous Tumours

8.1   Small cell carcinoma 8041/3
8.2   Tumour of probable wolffian origin 9110/1
8.3   Hepatoid carcinoma 8575/3
8.4   Myxoma 8840/0
8.5   Others

9   Gestational Trophoblastic Diseases

10   Soft Tissue Tumours Not Specific to Ovary

11   Malignant Lymphomas, Leukaemias and Plasmacytoma

12   Unclassified Tumours

13   Secondary (Metastatic) Tumours

14   Tumour-Like Lesions

Definitions and Explanatory Notes

1   Surface Epithelial-Stromal Tumours

Tumours composed of one or more of several distinctive types of epithelium and stroma in a variety of combinations.

These tumours are generally considered to arise from the surface epithelium of the ovary or its derivatives, the surface epithelial inclusion glands and the adjacent ovarian stroma. Other origins are possible for some of the subtypes, but unless another origin is unquestionable, the tumour is included in the surface epithelial-stromal category.

A form of surface epithelial-stromal tumour intermediate between one that is morphologically clearly benign and one that is obviously malignant has been termed a tumour "of borderline malignancy" or "of low malignant potential". This type of tumour has some, but not all, of the morphological features of malignancy. Those present include in varying combinations: nuclear abnormalities and mitotic activity that are generally intermediate between those of clearly benign and unquestionably malignant tumours of a similar cell type; stratification of the atypical epithelial cells accompanied by detachment of cellular clusters from their sites of origin in some tumours; and a lack of obvious invasion of the stromal component of the tumour. Tumours with epithelial cell proliferation or atypicality of a minor degree should be placed in the benign category.

The assessment of stromal invasion in serous and mucinous tumours is usually straightforward, but may be difficult in some cases in which penetration of the stroma by the tumour is orderly and unaccompanied by a recognizable stromal reaction. In such cases, confluence or very close approximation of glands or cysts lined by cells with a high degree of nuclear atypicality is tantamount to invasion. The distinction between borderline and invasive neoplasia is generally more difficult in cases of epithelial-stromal tumours of epithelial cell types other than serous and mucinous because of their rel-

ative rarity and controversy over their diagnostic criteria. An attempt
to differentiate borderline from invasive tumours within all cellular
subtypes is recommended, however, for purposes of investigation and
assessment of prognosis and therapy.

Benign, borderline and invasive components of any of the epithelial types discussed below may co-exist in a single specimen.

It must be emphasized that tumours of borderline malignancy, especially those in the serous category, occasionally implant on the
peritoneum, that such implants are invasive in a minority of the cases and that (occasionally) lymph node and (rarely) distant metastases
occur. In order that the histological diagnosis of the ovarian tumour
be morphologically objective and have prognostic significance, however, it must be based on an examination of the ovarian tumour itself
without consideration of whether spread beyond the ovary has oc-
curred. The practical validity of this diagnostic approach has been
demonstrated by the typically indolent course of borderline tumours
when they have spread beyond the ovary, the high survival rate of patients with peritoneal implants and the occasional spontaneous re-
gression of such implants. Another reason for evaluating the ovarian
tumour independently is the unresolved controversy whether the peritoneal "implants" associated with borderline tumours, especially
those in the serous category, are true implants in every case or reflect
synchronous primary neoplasia of the peritoneum in at least some
cases.

The descriptive prefixes "adeno-" and "cystadeno-" and the adjective "papillary" should be added to the designation of a surface epithelial-stromal tumour whenever appropriate. The suffix "-fibroma"
should be used when a tumour, with the exception of the Brenner tumour, is composed predominantly of benign-appearing stroma derived from the ovarian stroma. If the neoplastic epithelium is growing primarily on the outer surface of the ovary, the word "surface" is
an appropriate addition to the diagnostic term. The adjective indicat-
ing the epithelial cell type should generally be placed first among the
diagnostic words.

1.1   Serous tumours (Figs. 1–12)

*Tumours composed of epithelium resembling that of the fallopian
tube or in some cases the surface epithelium of the ovary.*

Ciliated cells are found in most benign serous tumours, in many
borderline tumours and in rare carcinomas. Psammoma bodies may

be present, at times in great profusion (Figs. 9, 11, 12), especially in carcinomas, but do not in themselves establish either the neoplastic nature of a process or the serous nature of a tumour. Carcinomas with extensive psammoma body formation and no more than moderate nuclear atypicality have been referred to as psammocarcinomas (Fig. 11). Serous neoplastic cells, particularly those in borderline tumours, may produce considerable mucin, which is almost entirely extracellular. Serous borderline tumours typically have well-developed papillary patterns; carcinomas are commonly papillary (Figs. 3, 6), but may have a predominantly glandular or diffuse pattern. Serous neoplastic cells may line intraovarian cysts or glands, the surface of the ovary or both.

Evidence exists that when serous borderline tumours have a "micropapillary" pattern, characterized by elongated stroma-poor or stroma-free papillae that emanate from a cyst wall or its polypoid extensions in a non-hierarchical manner (Fig. 6), or a cribriform pattern (Fig. 7), they are associated with invasive peritoneal implants more often than serous borderline tumours without such patterns and are therefore associated with a poorer prognosis.

Occasional serous borderline tumours exhibit foci of microinvasion of their stromal component, characterized by the presence of foci 3 mm or less in longest linear dimension and 10 sq. mm or less in area, containing tiny clusters of atypical cells lying in spaces that are not lined by endothelial cells (Fig. 8). These tumours are retained within the borderline category because their clinical behaviour appears to be much more similar to that of serous borderline tumours lacking this feature than to that of serous carcinomas.

1.2   Mucinous tumours, endocervical-like and intestinal types (Figs. 13–27)

Tumours, the epithelial element of which resembles endocervical (Figs. 13–16) or gastrointestinal epithelium (Figs. 17, 18). The latter almost always contains goblet cells, usually contains neuroendocrine cells (Fig. 18) and rarely contains Paneth cells.

The endocervical-like tumours have an epithelium that resembles that of the endocervix as well as that of the gastric pylorus and lacks goblet cells. The distinction between these tumours and those of the intestinal type is easy to make in benign and borderline cases, but is usually impossible and very likely clinically unimportant in cases of carcinoma. The distinction between the two subtypes is of greatest significance in borderline tumours. The endocervical-like borderline tumours have an architecture similar to that of serous borderline tumours, with papillae that contain abundant stroma and exhibit prominent cellular budding on their surfaces (Figs. 15, 16). These tumours may implant on the peritoneum and metastasize to lymph nodes; they are not associated with pseudomyxoma peritonei. In contrast, borderline mucinous tumours of intestinal type are either non-papillary or contain filiform, often branching papillae (Fig. 17). Some intestinal-type mucinous borderline tumours contain areas in which the cyst lining is obviously carcinomatous but is not associated with stromal invasion (Fig. 19). In such cases, it is recommended that the presence and extent of the intra-epithelial carcinoma be recorded in the diagnostic report and that extensive sampling of the specimen be performed to rule out stromal invasion.

Pseudomyxoma peritonei in the female is often associated with a mucinous cystic tumour of one or both ovaries with microscopic features that are usually consistent with intestinal-type borderline neoplasia but may appear benign or carcinomatous; the tumour typically contains areas of dissection of mucin into its stroma (pseudomyxoma ovarii) (Fig. 20). In some, and probably most such cases, a similar mucinous lesion of the appendix is also present. There is controversy whether the ovarian tumour is metastatic from the appendiceal tumour or whether both tumours are independently primary when they co-exist with pseudomyxoma peritonei. Nevertheless, the current practice has been to regard the ovarian tumour or tumours as primary for staging purposes in that situation. This approach to staging, if continued, must be undertaken with the realization that many of the ovarian tumours associated with pseudomyxoma peritonei may be metastatic and therefore do not reflect the biology of unquestionably primary ovarian mucinous borderline tumours of intestinal type.

The possibility of metastatic adenocarcinoma, particularly one of gastrointestinal or pancreatic origin, should be considered in cases of tumours having the microscopic features of a mucinous adenocarcinoma or even a mucinous borderline tumour of intestinal type in view of the remarkable degree of maturation of metastatic neoplastic epithelium that may occur within the ovary. Features suggesting a metastatic nature of the tumour in such cases include: bilaterality, the presence of surface implants, multinodularity, variable microscopical patterns from one nodule to another, extensive desmoplasia of the stroma and vascular space invasion. In some cases, metastasis cannot be excluded solely on the basis of examination of the ovarian tumour, and clinical information, operative findings and postoperative investigation may be required to solve the problem.

Rarely, one or more solid nodules are found in the wall of an ovarian mucinous cystic tumour that differ remarkably from the remainder of the tumour on microscopical examination. These nodules vary widely in their histologic features, ranging from sarcoma-like lesions containing epulis-like giant cells (Figs. 25, 26) to sarcoma, anaplastic carcinoma (Fig. 27) and carcinosarcoma.

1.3   Endometrioid tumours (Figs. 28–40)

Tumours with microscopical features resembling those of various tumour types that are encountered more commonly in the endometrium.

Although endometriosis, which is composed of epithelium and stroma of endometrial type, may have the gross features of a tumour, it lacks many characteristics of neoplasia and has been classified as a tumour-like lesion. A minority of endometrioid tumours can be shown to have arisen in endometriosis, but the demonstration of such an origin is not required for the diagnosis, and tumours other than endometrioid may develop in endometriosis.

The cells of endometrioid tumours may produce mucin, which is predominantly extracellular. Squamous differentiation of the neoplastic cells is common and, if present in an endometrioid carcinoma, warrants the diagnosis of endometrioid carcinoma with squamous differentiation; the squamous cells may have a benign or a malignant appearance (Figs. 28, 31). Endometrioid carcinomas may have a villoglandular pattern (Fig. 30), as sometimes seen in carcinomas of the endometrium; this pattern must be distinguished from the papillary patterns of other subtypes of surface-epithelial carcinoma such as serous and clear cell carcinomas.

A subset of endometrioid carcinomas has components that closely resemble granulosa cell and Sertoli or Sertoli-Leydig cell tumours (Figs. 32–34). Such tumours are usually identified by the finding of other patterns or cell types that are characteristic of endometrioid neoplasia and incompatible with a sex cord-stromal tumour. In difficult cases, the immunohistochemical positivity for epithelial membrane antigen and negativity for α-inhibin of endometrioid carcinomas and the converse findings in sex cord-stromal tumours are helpful in the differential diagnosis.

Endometrioid carcinoma of the ovary is often associated with a carcinoma of the endometrium that generally appears similar on microscopical examination. In such cases, it may be impossible to determine whether either or both tumours are primary, and the presence and extent of each should be recorded in the diagnosis. If the tumours are well differentiated and confined to the uterus and one or both ovaries, the prognosis is very good, strongly suggesting that the tumours are independently primary in such cases.

Endometrioid adenosarcomas (Figs. 35, 36) are characterized by benign-appearing to atypical glands, lined mostly by endometrioid, but occasionally other types of mullerian epithelium and distributed within a sarcomatous stroma that typically resembles low-grade endometrial stromal sarcoma or fibrosarcoma; the stromal component may contain heterologous elements.

Malignant mesodermal (mullerian) mixed tumours of the ovary are similar to those encountered more commonly in the uterine corpus, containing elements derived almost entirely from mesoderm. These tumours may be homologous or contain heterologous elements such as skeletal muscle, cartilage, osteoid and bone (Fig. 37). Unlike the immature teratoma, which almost always occurs in children or young women, the malignant mesodermal mixed tumour is encountered almost exclusively in menopausal or postmenopausal women. The cartilage that is found in heterologous mesodermal mixed tumours typically has bizarre nuclei similar to those that may be seen in chondrosarcomas (Fig. 37), whereas the cartilage in immature teratomas characteristically has a foetal appearance. The carcinomatous element of the mesodermal mixed tumour resembles various types within the surface epithelial category; in contrast, that of the immature teratoma typically has an embryonal appearance. Finally, the immature teratoma also contains structures of ectodermal (commonly neuroectodermal) and endodermal derivation.

Endometrioid stromal sarcomas closely resemble endometrial stromal sarcomas, but they also have a fibromatous component much more often than the latter (Figs. 38, 39). Occasionally, like its endometrial counterpart, the tumour contains foci of sex cord-like differentiation and simulates a granulosa cell tumour (Fig. 40). When they spread outside the ovary, endometrioid stromal sarcomas exhibit a characteristic tongue-like pattern of invasion.

It may be impossible to distinguish a primary endometrioid stromal sarcoma from a metastatic endometrial stromal sarcoma unless the uterus has been examined pathologically to exclude a similar tumour therein or unless the ovarian tumour can be shown to have arisen in endometriosis.

1.4   Clear cell tumours (Figs. 41–46)

Tumours composed of clear cells containing glycogen and resembling those of the renal cell carcinoma (Fig. 42), "hobnail" cells (characterized by scanty cytoplasm and large nuclei that project into a lumen) lining small cysts and tubules (Figs. 41, 43), occasionally, oxyphilic (Fig. 45), signet-ring (Fig. 46) or non-specific flat or cuboidal cells (Fig. 44) or a combination of these cell types.

Mucin secretion is often present within the cysts and tubules, but is absent intracellularly except within signet-ring cells. The patterns encountered include solid (Fig. 42), glandular, tubular, papillary (Fig. 43) and cystic (Figs. 41, 44) or combinations thereof.

On very rare occasions, a renal cell carcinoma metastasizes to the ovary and may be confused with a primary clear cell carcinoma that is composed entirely of clear cells. The clear cell carcinoma must also be distinguished from the yolk sac tumour, the dysgerminoma, steroid cell tumours and several other types of neoplasm.

1.5   Transitional cell tumours (Figs. 47–51)

Tumours containing epithelial cells resembling urothelial transitional cells.

The Brenner tumour (Figs. 47–50) is a transitional cell tumour in which mature urothelial-type cells lie in solid or cystic circumscribed nests within a predominantly fibromatous stroma in at least a component of the specimen. If the tumour also contains an atypical or cytologically malignant non-invasive component, it is borderline (Fig. 49). Because the small number of borderline tumours reported in the literature have not been proven to be malignant clinically, some investigators prefer the descriptive designation "proliferating" to "of borderline malignancy". Malignant Brenner tumours contain invasive transitional cell aggregates as well as benign nests (Fig. 50). Brenner tumours often contain mucinous epithelium, occasionally contain ciliated epithelium and may undergo squamous change.

Transitional cell carcinomas are malignant transitional cell tumours that do not have a component of benign Brenner tumour (Fig. 51). They are invasive tumours characterized by the presence of papillae lined by malignant cells of transitional type or nests of such cells in a fibrous or fibromatous stroma. Transitional cell carcinomas often contain a minor component of mucinous cells. These tumours are mixed with carcinomas of other surface epithelial cell types much more often than occurring in pure form.

Brenner tumours are occasionally encountered in association with a separate component of mucinous tumour. In such cases, the tumour should be reported according to the criteria established for the diagnosis of a mixed epithelial tumour (see below).

1.6   Squamous cell tumours

Tumours composed of squamous epithelial cells that are not clearly of germ cell origin.

Epidermoid cysts (Fig. 52) may be of germ cell or surface epithelial origin, but are classified as surface epithelial tumours unless obviously teratomatous elements are also present.

Most squamous cell carcinomas of the ovary belong in the germ cell category and arise in dermoid cysts. Squamous cell carcinomas in the epithelial-stromal category may originate in association with ovarian endometriosis or a Brenner tumour or may occur in pure form (without teratomatous elements).

1.7   Mixed epithelial tumours (specify components)
(Figs. 53–55)

Tumours composed of a mixture of two or more of the six types described above.

When less than 10% of a second or third type of epithelium is present, the tumour should be classified according to the predominant element. For example, endometrioid carcinomas, like similar carcinomas of the uterine corpus, occasionally contain foci of glands lined by mucin-filled epithelial cells, but their quantity is usually insufficient to warrant the diagnosis of a mixed epithelial tumour. In contrast, mucinous and Brenner tumours are occasionally admixed as separate components, with the minor component accounting for at least 10% of the entire neoplasm, qualifying for the diagnosis of a mixed epithelial tumour.

1.8   Undifferentiated carcinoma (Figs. 56, 57)

A malignant tumour of epithelial type that is too poorly differentiated to be placed in any of the preceding categories.

Although it may not be possible to establish the surface epithelial cell lineage of some tumours in this category, they are included therein in view of the frequently observed transitions between these tumours and clearly recognizable forms of epithelial cancer. Rare minor foci of differentiation, such as gland formation, psammoma body formation or mucin production, do not exclude the diagnosis of undifferentiated carcinoma.

Some undifferentiated carcinomas have neuroendocrine features resembling those of similar carcinomas encountered more often in other organs; the diagnosis can be confirmed by immunohistochemical staining. These tumours can be composed of cells with a moderate amount of cytoplasm or can resemble the oat-cell type of small cell carcinoma of the lung (Fig. 57). Tumours in the latter category must be differentiated from the small cell carcinoma that is usually associated with paraendocrine hypercalcaemia (see Sect. 8.1). Undifferentiated carcinomas with neuroendocrine features are usually mixed with an epithelial component of recognizable cell type such as mucinous, transitional or endometrioid (Fig. 57). If the tumour is of pure or almost pure small cell type, it should be classified as a primary neuroendocrine subtype of small cell carcinoma (see Sect. 8.1) after an extraovarian origin has been excluded.

2   Sex Cord-Stromal Tumours

Tumours containing granulosa cells, theca cells, collagen-producing stromal cells, Sertoli cells, Leydig cells and cells resembling the embryonic precursors of such cells, singly or in various combinations.

These tumours have also been designated "gonadal stromal tumours" on the disputed assumption that the gonadal sex cords are of stromal origin. The preferred generic term, sex cord-stromal tumours, is not intended to reflect a commitment to any one theory of gonadogenesis, but only acknowledges the presence in these tumours of two distinct categories of ovarian and testicular homologous cell types: granulosa and Sertoli cells (sex cord elements), and theca, Leydig and non-specific stromal-type cells (stromal elements).

2.1   Granulosa-stromal cell tumours

Tumours containing granulosa cells, theca cells or stromal cells resembling fibroblasts, or any combination of such cells.

2.1.1   *Granulosa cell tumours* (Figs. 58–66)

Tumours of ovarian cell types containing more than a minor component of granulosa cells (10% or more).

Granulosa cell tumours have been divided into two subtypes: the adult, which occurs in adults in over 90% of cases; and the juvenile, which is much rarer and occurs in the first three decades of life in over 90% of cases.

The adult granulosa cell tumour is typically associated with menstrual irregularities or postmenopausal bleeding and generally has an indolent course, with a 10-year survival rate of 90%, but only about a 70% survival at 30 years because of late recurrences.

The cells of the adult granulosa cell tumour (Figs. 58–62) typically have round, oval or angular, pale, often grooved nuclei and may be arranged in a variety of patterns, including follicular (microfollicular and macrofollicular) (Fig. 58), trabecular (Fig. 59), insular, gyriform, watered-silk and diffuse (Fig. 61). A mixture of patterns often exists in a single tumour. Theca cells are often present in addition to granulosa cells; either cell type may be luteinized (i.e. contain abundant cytoplasm and have a morphological appearance similar to that of cells of the corpus luteum) (Fig. 62). The microfollicular pattern is characterized by the presence of distinctive Call-Exner bodies (Figs. 58, 60).

The juvenile granulosa cell tumour (Figs. 63–66) is typically associated with isosexual precocity. The survival rate is approximately 90%, and late recurrences are rare. The tumour cells are usually arranged in nodules, which may be solid or punctured by follicles that are generally of moderate size, vary in shape (Fig. 63) and contain mucicarminophilic fluid (Fig. 66); Call-Exner bodies are absent or rare. Theca cells are often present (Fig. 65). The tumour cells are usually luteinized, with considerable eosinophilic (Fig. 64) or lipid-rich cytoplasm (Fig. 65); the nuclei generally are darker than those of the adult granulosa cell tumour and lack grooves (Fig. 64). Occasionally, the nuclei are pleomorphic, sometimes resulting in an erroneous diagnosis of a malignant germ cell tumour.

Adenocarcinomas with small, uniform glands, particularly microglandular forms of endometrioid adenocarcinoma, may superficially resemble microfollicular adult granulosa cell tumours and are sometimes misdiagnosed as such. A similar problem in differential diagnosis exists for undifferentiated carcinomas, which may resemble superficially diffuse adult granulosa cell tumours. A diagnostic feature of the adult granulosa cell tumour that is more specific than its characteristic patterns is the appearance of its nuclei; they may be either angular, with their long axes oriented haphazardly, or round or oval and uniform; although mitoses may be numerous, the nuclei are typically pale, lacking the pleomorphism and hyperchromatism of those of most adenocarcinomas and undifferentiated carcinomas. Rare granulosa cell tumours, however, contain bizarre nuclei similar to those seen in the symplastic leiomyoma of the uterus. The frequent presence of nuclear grooves in granulosa cells is additionally helpful in the differential diagnosis. Microfollicular adult granulosa cell tumours must also be distinguished from primary and metastatic insular carcinoid tumours. Diffuse adult granulosa cell tumours must be differentiated from primary endometrioid stromal sarcomas and metastatic endometrial stromal sarcomas. Immunohistochemical staining of granulosa cells for α-inhibin is particularly helpful in the rare cases in which the above differential diagnoses are difficult on the basis of routine staining.

2.1.2   Tumours in thecoma–fibroma group

Tumours forming a continuous spectrum from those composed entirely of cells resembling fibroblasts and producing collagen to those containing a predominance of cells resembling theca cells.

2.1.2.1   Thecoma (Figs. 67–69)

A stromal tumour, many cells of which resemble theca cells, lutein cells or both; cells resembling fibroblasts are usually present as well.

The tumour has been divided into two subtypes, the typical and luteinized forms. The typical thecoma is composed of sheets or nodules of large, ill-defined cells with moderate to abundant pale cytoplasm, which is usually rich in lipid, alternating with a variable component of spindle cells that have produced collagen (Fig. 67). Typical thecomas are oestrogenic in almost all cases. Luteinized thecomas contain clusters of sharply defined steroid-type cells with moderate to abundant eosinophilic to lipid-rich vacuolated cytoplasm on a background of a fibromatous or typical thecomatous proliferation (Fig. 68). Luteinized thecomas are oestrogenic in half the cases and androgenic in approximately 10% of cases. A rare form of luteinized thecoma, in which there may be marked mitotic activity, is associated with sclerosing peritonitis. Another rare tumour has the general features of luteinized thecoma, but in addition contains crystals of

Reinke in one or more of its steroid-type cells; this tumour has been called "stromal Leydig cell tumour" (Fig. 69).

Thecomas are almost always benign. They should be differentiated from diffuse granulosa cell tumours; reticulin staining, which reveals an abundance of fibrils investing individual thecoma cells and relatively few fibrils within aggregates of granulosa cells, is often helpful in the differential diagnosis, but in some cases demonstrates an intermediate pattern, which is of no diagnostic value.

2.1.2.2   Fibroma (Fig. 70)

A stromal tumour composed of spindle cells producing abundant collagen.

The fibroma may have a pattern of intersecting fascicles (Fig. 70) or a storiform pattern. Some fibromas are markedly oedematous; such tumours are more apt to be associated with ascites or ascites and hydrothorax (Demons-Meigs syndrome) than fibromas containing little intercellular fluid. The fibroma may have considerable intracellular lipid, but is rarely associated with steroid hormone production. Fibromas are common in the basal cell naevus syndrome, in which they are typically bilateral and calcified. It is possible that an occasional fibroma is derived from the fibroblasts of non-specific fibrous tissue within the ovary rather than from ovarian stromal cells.

2.1.2.3   Cellular fibroma (Fig. 71)

A fibroma characterized by closely packed nuclei and scanty collagen.

Mitotic figures generally range from 1 to 3 per 10 high-power fields, and nuclear atypicality is absent to minimal. The tumour may recur, particularly if it has ruptured or is adherent; recurrence may not be clinically evident until 10 or more years postoperatively.

2.1.2.4   Fibrosarcoma

A fibroblastic tumour that typically has more than 3 mitotic figures per 10 high-power fields as well as significant nuclear atypicality.

2.1.2.5   Stromal tumour with minor sex cord elements

A tumour in the thecoma–fibroma group that contains small nests of cells or tubules of sex cord derivation that account for less than 10% of the neoplastic tissue.

2.1.2.6   Sclerosing stromal tumour (Figs. 72, 73)

A tumour characterized by cellular pseudolobules composed of a disorderly admixture of collagen-producing fibroblasts and generally lipid-rich lutein cells with shrunken nuclei; the pseudolobules are separated by hypocellular dense or edematous fibrous tissue and may be highly vascular.

The tumour occurs in young women and may be oestrogenic or rarely androgenic, especially during pregnancy.

2.1.2.7   Stromal luteoma (see Sect. 2.6.1)

This tumour is best classified as an identifiable subtype of steroid cell tumour.

2.1.2.8   Unclassified

A tumour with features intermediate between those of a fibroma and those of a thecoma.

2.1.2.9   Others

This category includes the signet-ring stromal tumour (Fig. 74), in which many of the cells have nuclei displaced by a large, round, fluid-filled vacuole that does not contain fat, glycogen or mucin. This tumour must be differentiated from rare granulosa cell tumours containing similar vacuoles as well as a wide variety of ovarian tumours with vacuoles that appear similar on routine staining but are generally shown to contain other substances such as mucin or lipid on special staining.

2.2   Sertoli-stromal cell tumours, androblastomas

Tumours containing in pure form or in various combinations Sertoli cells, cells resembling rete epithelial cells, cells resembling fibroblasts and Leydig cells in variable degrees of differentiation.

The designation "androblastoma" is preferred by some investigators, but it has the confusing connotations of an origin from male "blastema", for which there is little evidence, and of androgen production even though the tumour is often non-functioning and occasionally oestrogenic.

2.2.1   Well differentiated

2.2.1.1   Sertoli cell tumour (tubular androblastoma) (Figs. 75, 76)

A tumour composed entirely or almost entirely of Sertoli cells forming well-defined tubules.

The tubules may have lumens or be solid like those of the prepubertal testis; the cells may be arranged in broad trabeculae (Fig. 76). The tumour cells can contain lipid in variable and occasionally large quantities (Fig. 75). Leydig cells may be present in small numbers. The tumour may have oestrogenic or occasionally androgenic manifestations.

Sertoli cell tumours must be distinguished from tubular forms of certain other tumours such as endometrioid carcinoma, carcinoid tumour, struma ovarii and Krukenberg tumour.

2.2.1.2   Sertoli-Leydig cell tumour (Fig. 77)

A tumour containing more than a small component of Leydig cells in addition to well-defined tubules.

The tumour is often androgenic and occasionally oestrogenic.

2.2.1.3   Leydig cell tumour (see Sect. 2.6.2)

This tumour is best classified as an identifiable subtype of steroid cell tumour.

2.2.2   Sertoli-Leydig cell tumour of intermediate differentiation
(Figs. 78, 79)

A tumour in which immature Sertoli cells are typically arranged diffusely, in islands, in cords resembling testicular embryonic sex cords or in several other epithelial-type patterns. Well-differentiated tubules may be present additionally. Non-specific-appearing stromal cells and well-differentiated Leydig cells are also identifiable.

2.2.3   Sertoli-Leydig cell tumour, poorly differentiated
(sarcomatoid) (Fig. 80)

A tumour composed largely of tissue resembling a sarcoma, but also containing recognizable Sertoli cells and Leydig cells. Rarely, the Sertoli cell element is the poorly differentiated component.

2.2.4   Retiform (Figs. 81, 82)

A tumour that resembles the rete testis in its architecture and cell type.

The tumour is rarely seen in pure form, being almost always admixed with other types of Sertoli-stromal cell tumour. Some retiform tumours closely simulate surface epithelial-stromal tumours in the borderline and malignant categories, especially those in the serous group (Fig. 82).

Heterologous elements, mainly mucinous epithelium of gastrointestinal type (Fig. 83), sometimes accompanied by carcinoid tumourlets, and occasionally cartilage or skeletal muscle within a sarcomatous component have been seen in about 20% of Sertoli-Leydig cell tumours in the intermediate, poorly differentiated or retiform categories. The heterologous elements are not considered to reflect teratomatous differentiation of a germ cell tumour in view of the limited variability of the heterologous differentiation and the absence of gonadal differentiation in any ovarian tumour that is unquestionably teratomatous.

2.3   Sex cord tumour with annular tubules (Figs. 84, 85)

A sex cord tumour characterized by the presence of simple and complex ring-shaped tubules.

The simple tubules have a central round hyaline deposit around which a solid tubule with peripheral nuclei and central cytoplasm has rotated. The complex tubules form larger aggregates in which a solid tubule winds around multiple round hyaline deposits (Fig. 84). Focal differentiation into both typical Sertoli cell tumour and typical microfollicular granulosa cell tumour is sometimes observed. Occasional tumour cells have been shown to contain bundles of Charcot-Bottcher filaments, which are characteristic constituents of normal Sertoli cells. The sex cord tumour with annular tubules occurs in two situations – more often as a large solitary tumour, which is frequently oestrogenic and occasionally progestagenic, and less often in the form of multiple, often calcified tumourlets (Fig. 85), which are occasionally oestrogenic, in patients with the Peutz-Jeghers syndrome. The solitary tumour is malignant in about one quarter of cases; the tumourlets are benign.

2.4   Gynandroblastoma

A very rare tumour in which aggregates of granulosa cells containing typical Call-Exner bodies co-exist with hollow tubules lined by Sertoli cells.

The term is only morphological and does not imply the presence of both oestrogenic and androgenic manifestations. Other combinations of granulosa-stromal and Sertoli-stromal cell tumour also exist, e.g. intermediate Sertoli-Leydig cell tumour and juvenile granulosa cell tumour.

2.5   Unclassified sex cord-stromal tumour

A tumour in which sex cord or stromal elements or both are present but cannot be specifically identified as either ovarian or testicular in type because of indeterminate or poor differentiation.

2.6   Steroid (lipid) cell tumours (Figs. 86–90)

Tumours composed exclusively or almost exclusively of cells that resemble Leydig, lutein and adrenal cortical cells.

Those tumours of established ovarian stromal or lutein cell origin are designated "stromal luteoma"; those composed of steroid-type cells containing crystals of Reinke as Leydig cell tumours; and those that cannot be placed in either of the above two categories as "steroid cell tumours, not otherwise specified" (NOS), or "unclassified". Diagnosis of the first two subtypes depends on the topography of the tumour (i.e. an intrastromal or hilar location) and the presence or absence of crystals of Reinke.

2.6.1   Stromal luteoma (Figs. 86, 87)

A steroid cell tumour without crystals surrounded by a rim of ovarian stroma.

Occasionally, degenerative changes result in the formation of spaces containing red blood cells (Fig. 87); in such cases, the tumour is sometimes mistaken for a vascular tumour. The stromal luteoma is usually accompanied by stromal hyperthecosis (focal luteinization of the stroma uninvolved by the tumour) and is typically oestrogenic.

2.6.2   Leydig cell tumour (Fig. 88)

A tumour composed exclusively of Leydig cells.

Either a predominantly hilar location of a steroid cell tumour or the intracellular presence of crystals of Reinke or both warrant the diagnosis of Leydig cell tumour. A hilar location with or without crystal-containing cells indicates a Leydig cell tumour of hilar type (hilus cell tumour); a Leydig cell tumour surrounded by ovarian stroma is a Leydig cell tumour, non-hilar type. In some cases in which the tumour occupies both stroma and hilus, it is impossible to establish the site of origin. Leydig cell tumours are typically androgenic.

2.6.3   Steroid cell tumour, unclassified (not otherwise specified)
        (Figs. 89, 90)

*A large steroid cell tumour that has lost its topographic features and
lacks crystals of Reinke.*

   Tumours in this category have also been referred to as "lipid cell
tumours" and "lipoid cell tumours", but these terms are inappropriate
because of their lack of specificity and the absence of intracellular
lipid in one quarter of the cases. Steroid cell tumours, unclassified,
are usually virilizing but may be oestrogenic or non-functioning. Occasionally, they are accompanied by elevated levels of corticosteroids
or clinically recognizable Cushing syndrome. These associations
gave rise to the formerly used terms "adrenal rest tumour" and "adre-
nal-like tumour". Such tumours, however, are now generally considered to be of gonadal cell origin, with ectopic production of adreno-
corticosteroid hormones. About one quarter of steroid cell tumours,
unclassified, are malignant. It may be difficult to distinguish between
benign and malignant forms in the absence of metastasis, but increas-
ing age, the presence of Cushing syndrome, a diameter of 7 cm or
greater, nuclear atypia, a mitotic count of 2 or more per 10 high-power fields and the presence of necrosis and haemorrhage favour malignancy.

3   Germ Cell Tumours

*A broad category of tumours derived from germ cells, ranging from
undifferentiated forms to tumours with an extra-embryonic appearance to tumours containing immature or mature tissues or both that
represent two or more of the three embryonic layers (ectoderm, mesoderm and endoderm) or a single layer exclusive of mesoderm.*

3.1   Dysgerminoma (Figs. 91–94)

*A tumour composed of large, rounded, typically clear cells that re-
semble primordial germ cells both morphologically and on special
and immunohistochemical staining.*

   The cells are usually arranged diffusely (Fig. 91) or in islands or
strands separated by variable amounts of fibrous tissue infiltrated by
lymphocytes; granulomas, which may contain Langhans giant cells,
are often present (Fig. 93). The nuclei of the tumour cells are central

and imperfectly rounded and contain one to four prominent nucleoli (Fig. 92); the cytoplasm contains glycogen, the presence of which may be of diagnostic aid. Immunohistochemical staining is positive for placental-like alkaline phosphatase, neuron-specific enolase, vimentin and occasionally cytokeratin (usually focally).

Five to ten percent of dysgerminomas contain syncytiotrophoblast cells (Fig. 94), which secrete chorionic gonadotropin (hCG) and can account for elevation of this hormone in the serum and occasional oestrogenic or androgenic manifestations.

3.2   Yolk sac tumour (endodermal sinus tumour)
    (Figs. 95–103)

A tumour of many epithelial patterns, the most common of which is reticular, characterized by a network of spaces lined by primitive cells that are typically positive immunohistochemically for alpha fetoprotein (αFP).

In many cases, single rounded, occasionally elongated papillae containing a solitary central blood vessel (Schiller-Duval bodies) protrude into the spaces (Figs. 95, 96) and have been likened to the endodermal sinuses of the rat placenta, which are of yolk sac origin. The designation "endodermal sinus tumour" is optimally restricted to yolk sac tumours with this pattern. Sometimes, a more complex papillary pattern is present. A solid arrangement of tumour cells, which may be perforated by small slit-like spaces, may be seen, usually only focally, and may resemble a dysgerminoma on routine staining (Fig. 98); the lymphocytic infiltration typical of the latter tumour, however, is absent. The nuclei of typical yolk sac tumours are usually poorly differentiated; the cytoplasm often contains hyaline bodies (Fig. 97).

A variant of yolk sac tumour, which is almost always present only focally, is the polyvesicular vitelline tumour, characterized by numerous vesicles resembling embryonic yolk sac vesicles, separated by mesenchymal tissue (Fig. 99). Occasionally, the vesicles divide eccentrically into a large component lined by flattened cells, simulating the vestigial primary yolk sac vesicle of the embryo, and a small component lined by taller epithelium, resembling the secondary yolk sac vesicle (Fig. 100). The latter develops into the gastrointestinal tract and its appendages in the normal embryo.

The glandular variant of yolk sac tumour has two main subtypes, one of which is composed of cells consistent with primitive intestinal epithelium growing in a cribriform pattern (Fig. 101), and the other of which is better differentiated and resembles endometrioid adeno-carcinoma of the usual or secretory type in routine sections (Fig. 102). The latter tumour has been referred to as an "endometrioid-like" yolk sac tumour. The hepatoid variant of yolk sac tumour closely resembles hepatocellular carcinoma (Fig. 103). The diagnosis of these variants can be confirmed by staining for αFP.

Very rare yolk sac tumours are not of germ cell origin but develop within surface epithelial-stromal tumours.

3.3   Embryonal carcinoma (Fig. 104)

A tumour composed of epithelial cells resembling those of the embryonic germ disc and growing in one or more of several patterns – glandular, tubular, papillary and solid.

This tumour, which is commonly encountered in the testis, is very rare in the ovary, where the yolk sac tumour accounts for almost all the highly malignant non-teratomatous germ cell tumours. The embryonal carcinoma often contains scattered syncytiotrophoblast cells and may also contain foci of yolk sac differentiation. The tumour is positive immunohistochemically for placental-like alkaline phosphatase, cytokeratin, Ber H2 (CD30) and usually hCG, but is negative for epithelial membrane antigen.

3.4   Polyembryoma

A very rare tumour composed predominantly or exclusively of embryoid bodies resembling normal early embryos.

3.5   Choriocarcinoma (Fig. 105)

A rare tumour composed of both cytotrophoblast and syncytiotrophoblast.

The tumour is much more commonly present as a component of a mixed germ cell tumour than as a pure neoplasm. Besides being of germ cell origin, an ovarian choriocarcinoma may arise in an ovarian pregnancy or may have spread to the ovary from another site in the genital tract. Very rare choriocarcinomas are not of germ cell origin but develop within surface epithelial-stromal tumours.

3.6   Teratomas

Tumours composed of tissues resembling derivatives of two or three of the embryonic layers (ectoderm, mesoderm, endoderm) or of a single layer other than mesoderm.

The structures present may be immature (embryonal), mature (foetal or adult) or both. In occasional cases, the differentiation is purely or mostly monodermal, with the exclusive, predominant or grossly recognizable presence of a specialized type of tissue.

3.6.1   Immature teratoma (Fig. 106)

A teratoma that contains embryonal tissue.

Mature tissue is usually present as well. The predominant embryonal tissue is almost always neuroectodermal. Although most immature teratomas are predominantly solid, an occasional one is predominantly cystic. Immature teratomas are graded according to the amount of embryonal tissue they contain, which correlates with their prognosis.

3.6.2   Mature teratoma

A teratoma composed exclusively of foetal or adult structures or both.

3.6.2.1   Solid (Fig. 107)

It is important to differentiate between mature and immature solid teratomas because the former are almost invariably benign, while the latter are often clinically malignant. The occasional presence of implants of mature glia or, rarely, mature tissue of other types on the peritoneum may be associated with either an immature or mature solid teratoma, but per se does not warrant a diagnosis of malignancy.

3.6.2.2   Cystic (dermoid cyst) (Fig. 108)

A mature teratoma characterized by a predominance of one or a few cysts lined by epidermis, accompanied by its appendages.

The tumour often contains mature neuroectodermal derivatives as well; elements of both endodermal and mesodermal origin are also found in most cases. Occasionally, respiratory epithelium or glia forms a portion of the lining and, very rarely, the entire lining of a mature cystic teratoma.

3.6.2.3   With secondary tumour (specify type)

A wide variety of benign and malignant tumours may arise from the constituents of a mature cystic teratoma. Squamous cell carcinoma is the usual form of malignant change (Fig. 109); adenocarcinomas and sarcomas are much less common; other tumours, including malignant melanoma, are rare. Highly specialized tumours that may arise in association with a dermoid cyst are discussed in the section on monodermal teratomas (Sect. 3.6.3).

3.6.2.4   Foetiform teratoma (homunculus)

A rare form of mature teratoma resembling externally a foetus.

It may have a rudimentary head, trunk and extremities. The tumour must be differentiated from a foetus in foetu, which does not occupy the ovary and contains a much wider variety of organs and tissues than the foetiform teratoma.

3.6.3   Monodermal

3.6.3.1   Struma ovarii (Figs. 110–112)

A teratoma in which thyroid tissue is exclusively or almost exclusively present or forms a grossly recognizable component of a teratoma.

The tumour commonly has a predominant or exclusive appearance of a follicular adenoma or other type of tumour seen in the thyroid gland (Fig. 110) rather than that of normal thyroid parenchyma. A small number of strumas resembling thyroid tumours are malignant on microscopic examination (Fig. 111), and some of these have been clinically malignant as well. Rare examples of struma with a tubular pattern or a predominance of clear cells or oxyphilic cells may mimic other ovarian tumours with similar patterns or cell types (Figs. 112). Immunohistochemical staining for thyroglobulin facilitates the diagnosis of struma in such cases. Rarely, strumas cause or contribute to the development of hyperthyroidism.

3.6.3.2   Carcinoid tumours

Tumours with extensive components of neuroendocrine cells; most subtypes resemble carcinoid tumours of the gastrointestinal tract.

A primary carcinoid tumour may be pure or relatively pure or may be part of a more complex teratoma.

3.6.3.2.1 Insular carcinoid tumour (Figs. 113)

A tumour containing discrete islands of neoplastic cells with or without acinus formation and resembling the midgut type of intestinal carcinoid tumour.

The tumour may be associated with the carcinoid syndrome in the absence of metastatic disease.

3.6.3.2.2 Trabecular carcinoid tumour (Fig. 114)

A tumour containing trabeculae or ribbons of neoplastic cells and resembling a hindgut carcinoid tumour.

This tumour rarely produces clinically significant amounts of hormone.

Rare carcinoid tumours have unusual patterns, such as a solid tubular pattern that resembles a Sertoli cell tumour on routine staining. Immunohistochemical staining for chromogranin, synaptophysin and neuron-specific enolase is often helpful in confirming the diagnosis of carcinoid in difficult cases.

Both insular and trabecular carcinoid tumours must be distinguished from metastatic carcinoid tumours, which, in contrast to the former, are commonly bilateral. In metastatic cases, the primary tumour may be occult.

3.6.3.3   Strumal carcinoid tumour (Figs. 115–117)

A tumour composed of thyroid-type tissue intimately associated with ribbons and islands of carcinoid tumour.

The carcinoid component, which is most often trabecular, typically invades the strumal component, with neuroendocrine cells replacing the follicular lining cells. The tumour is rarely associated with evidence of hyperfunction of the strumal component or the carcinoid syndrome.

3.6.3.4   Goblet cell carcinoid tumour (Figs. 118, 119)

A carcinoid tumour containing goblet cells as well as neuroendocrine cells, resembling the goblet cell carcinoid tumour of the appendix.
Well-differentiated forms are composed of small, discrete, rounded nests and glands containing goblet cells and neuroendocrine cells. Individual tumour cells may contain both mucin and neuroendocrine granules. In poorly differentiated areas, there may be a diffuse arrangement of signet-ring cells resembling a Krukenberg tumour. Goblet cell carcinoid tumours may also be metastatic from the appendix.

3.6.3.5   Neuroectodermal tumours (specify type)

Neuroectodermal tumours include well-differentiated forms such as the ependymoma (Fig. 120), poorly differentiated tumours that resemble primitive neuroectodermal tumours of the central nervous system and soft tissues, and anaplastic forms that resemble glioblastoma multiforme.

3.6.3.6   Sebaceous tumours

These tumours almost always arise in the wall of a dermoid cyst and simulate various forms of cutaneous sebaceous gland tumours.

3.6.3.7   Others

This category includes hormone-secreting pituitary-type tumours, which may be associated with endocrine manifestations, and retinal anlage tumours.

3.7   Mixed germ cell tumours (Fig. 121)

Tumours consisting of a mixture of specified types of germ cell tumour.

Each component should be identified in the diagnosis and quantified as far as possible, especially if the tumour is malignant.

4   Gonadoblastoma (Figs. 122-124)

A tumour composed of two main cell types, large germ cells, which are generally similar to those of the dysgerminoma and seminoma, and small cells, which resemble immature Sertoli cells; in addition, the stroma usually contains cells that resemble Leydig cells but lack crystals of Reinke.

The two main cell types usually grow within discrete solid aggregates that typically contain rounded hyaline masses composed of basement membrane material (Fig. 122) and often contain foci of calcification (Fig. 123). The germ cells and Sertoli-like cells occasionally grow diffusely. In some cases, the germ cells transgress the margins of the mixed-cellular aggregates and grow as a germinoma (dysgerminoma or seminoma) (Fig. 124) or, much less often, as another form of germ cell tumour. Some gonadoblastomas are identified as residual small foci within or adjacent to a germinoma or another type of germ cell tumour.

Gonadoblastomas arise almost exclusively in patients with dysgenetic ovaries or testes or both. Most of the patients are phenotypic females who are usually virilized to a variable extent, and almost all have chromatin-negative nuclei and a Y-chromosome or at least a specific fragment of it. Very rarely, the tumour occurs in an apparently normal fertile female.

5   Germ Cell-Sex Cord-Stromal Tumour
of Non-gonadoblastoma Type (Fig. 125)

A very rare tumour occurring in otherwise normal ovaries, composed of an admixture of germ cells and sex cord elements, with additional stromal derivatives in some cases.

The tumour typically lacks rounded hyaline masses and calcification; its germ cells may resemble those of the dysgerminoma or may appear more differentiated. The tumour arises in individuals with a

normal karyotype and normal sexual development and may be oestrogenic. In some cases, pure germ cell neoplasia develops within the tumour and may be the predominant neoplastic element in the specimen.

6   Tumours of Rete Ovarii (Fig. 126)

These very rare tumours arise in the hilus and range from adenomas
and cystadenomas to cystadenocarcinomas. Unlike typical serous
cystadenomas, rete cystadenomas have no or very few cilia and have
shallow crevices in their walls (Fig. 126). They often contain a layer
of hypertrophied smooth muscle, hyperplastic hilus cells or both in
their walls. The hilus cell hyperplasia may be associated with viriliza-
tion.

7   Mesothelial Tumours

Adenomatoid tumours arise very rarely in the ovarian hilus
(Fig. 127). Exceptionally, malignant epithelial mesotheliomas are entirely or mostly confined to the ovarian surface and may even invade
and replace underlying ovarian tissue. The ovaries are also commonly involved in cases of diffuse malignant mesothelioma of the peritoneum.

8   Tumours of Uncertain Origin
and Miscellaneous Primary Tumours

8.1   Small cell carcinoma (Figs. 128–131)

Ovarian small cell carcinomas are of two types – one that is usually
associated with paraendocrine hypercalcaemia and has been referred
to as "small cell carcinoma, hypercalcaemic type" and the other that
has neuroendocrine features and has been designated "small cell carcinoma, pulmonary type"; evidence suggests that the latter belongs in
the surface epithelial-stromal subcategory of undifferentiated carcinoma (see Sect. 1.8). The small cell carcinoma of hypercalcaemic
type almost always occurs in patients in the second to fourth decades
and is characterized by the formation of follicle-like spaces (Fig. 128)

and the presence of nuclei that contain easily visible nucleoli (Fig. 129). Despite the designation "small cell carcinoma", areas composed of large cells with abundant eosinophilic cytoplasm and nuclei containing prominent nucleoli (Fig. 130) are often encountered and occasionally predominate in the tumour. Mucin-filled cells with either benign or malignant-appearing nuclei may also be present (Fig. 131). Dense core granules are absent or rare on ultrastructural examination; the tumour is typically diploid on flow cytometry. Paraendocrine hypercalcaemia is present in approximately two thirds of cases, but paraneoplastic and other paraendocrine manifestations have not been reported.

The small cell carcinoma of pulmonary type occurs mainly in older women in association with a surface epithelial-stromal tumour and is characterized by nuclei that are often molded, have finely stippled chromatin and lack easily discernible nucleoli. Tumours of this cell type originating in the lung and elsewhere are usually aneuploid, are rarely associated with paraendocrine hypercalcaemia and often have other paraendocrine and paraneoplastic manifestations.

8.2   Tumour of probable wolffian origin (Figs. 132, 133)

A tumour characterized by a variety of epithelial patterns – diffuse, sieve-like, solid-tubular and hollow-tubular, combinations of which are typically present within individual tumours.

The neoplastic cells generally have a bland appearance, and the tumour is usually benign.

8.3   Hepatoid carcinoma

An αFP-positive tumour that resembles to a variable extent a hepatocellular carcinoma, but is not of germ cell origin.

An occasional admixture with serous carcinoma provides strong evidence of a surface epithelial origin. The tumour can be distinguished from the hepatoid yolk sac tumour by its less striking resemblance to hepatocellular carcinoma and by the different associated patterns or cell types of the two tumours. Moreover, the hepatoid carcinoma typically occurs at an older age than the hepatoid yolk sac tumour.

8.4   Myxoma (Fig. 134)

A tumour characterized by bland-appearing spindle and stellate cells distributed within an abundant, well-vascularized myxoid background.

Lipoblasts are absent. Small foci of fibromatous tissue or smooth muscle may be present. The tumour is usually benign but can recur late.

8.5   Others

This category includes tumours resembling adenoid cystic carcinoma and basal cell carcinoma, many of which are probably of surface epithelial lineage, as well as the very rare oncocytoma, an oxyphilic tumour in which the cytoplasm contains prominent granules.

9   Gestational Trophoblastic Disease

Rare hydatidiform moles and choriocarcinomas arise as a result of ectopic ovarian pregnancy. Choriocarcinoma can also be of germ cell origin or metastatic from the genital tract.

10   Soft Tissue Tumours Not Specific to the Ovary

These tumours should be classified according to the WHO Histological Typing of Soft Tissue Tumours[1].

11   Malignant Lymphomas (Figs. 135, 136), Leukaemias and Plasmacytoma

Lymphomas and leukaemias may involve the ovary and grow diffusely or in the form of well-defined nests and cords, simulating the patterns of a carcinoma or dysgerminoma (Figs. 135, 136). Lymphoma is occasionally primary in the ovary and is curable in a minority of

---

[1]Weiss SW (1994) Histological typing of soft tissue tumours, 2nd edn. Springer, Berlin Heidelberg New York.

such cases. Burkitt lymphoma is a type that commonly presents with ovarian involvement. Very rarely, a leukaemic tumour, such as a granulocytic sarcoma or a plasmacytoma, presents as an ovarian tumour.

12 Unclassified Tumours

Primary ovarian tumours that cannot be placed in any of the categories described above.

13 Secondary (Metastatic) Tumours

Secondary tumours, which may be of a wide variety of types, account for 5%–15% of malignant ovarian tumours encountered during exploration of an adnexal mass. Carcinomas of the gastrointestinal tract, genital tract and breast and tumours of the haematopoietic system account for most of these neoplasms.

The Krukenberg tumour has a distinctive appearance characterized by the presence of mucin-filled signet-ring cells accompanied by a reactive proliferation of the ovarian stroma (Fig. 137). This tumour is usually secondary to a gastric carcinoma, but may originate in other organs in which mucinous carcinomas arise, including the breast and intestine. Occasionally, the tumour has a glandular, cystic or tubular pattern, any of which may predominate. The stroma is often oedematous or myxoid.

Very rarely, a tumour with the pattern of a Krukenberg tumour appears to be primary in the ovary. Either a prolonged disease-free follow-up period (10 years or longer) or an exhaustive autopsy that fails to reveal an extra-ovarian primary tumour is essential for the diagnosis.

The most common problem in the differentiation of metastatic and primary ovarian tumours is the distinction between a metastatic intestinal carcinoma and a primary endometrioid or mucinous carcinoma. A confusing feature in some metastatic mucinous carcinomas is maturation of the epithelial linings of cysts to the extent that they are difficult to distinguish from the linings of cysts in borderline mucinous tumours and even mucinous cystadenomas (Fig. 138). The much higher frequency of bilaterality of the metastatic intestinal tumour and its distinctive gross and histologic features (Fig 139) almost always lead to a correct diagnosis based on routine staining.

In difficult cases, immunohistochemical staining may be helpful in the differential diagnosis; primary ovarian carcinomas are typically positive for human alveolar macrophage (HAM)-56 and cytokeratin-7 and negative for cytokeratin-20; the converse is true for metastatic intestinal carcinoma.

Carcinoid tumours that have metastasized to the ovary are important to be aware of because the primary tumour may be clinically inapparent and the metastatic tumour can be confused with several types of primary ovarian tumour, including carcinoid tumour, granulosa cell tumour and Sertoli cell tumour.

It may be difficult to distinguish metastatic tumours of genital tract and breast origin from independent primary tumours of the ovary that have similar appearances. Tumour distribution, gross and microscopic features, immunohistochemical staining, ploidy analysis and molecular genetic studies have been used in these differential diagnoses.

14   Tumour-like Lesions

14.1   Solitary follicle cyst

A follicle that enlarges after failing to undergo ovulation, rarely exceeding 8 cm in diameter.

The cyst wall consists of granulosa cells, theca cells or both; either or both cell types may be luteinized.

14.2   Multiple follicle cysts (polycystic ovarian disease, sclerocystic ovaries) (Figs. 140, 141)

Bilateral ovarian enlargement by numerous slightly enlarged follicles that have failed to ovulate.

Follicular hyperthecosis and sclerosis of the outer cortex are additional features.

14.3   Large solitary luteinized follicle cyst of pregnancy and puerperium (Fig. 142)

A generally very large cyst diagnosed during pregnancy or at the first puerperal visit and characterized by foci of bizarre nuclei in the luteinized granulosa cells or theca cells within the cyst wall.

14.4   Hyperreactio luteinalis
(multiple luteinized follicle cysts) (Fig. 143)

Bilateral ovarian enlargement, which may be marked, characterized by multiple extensively luteinized follicles and marked stromal congestion and edema.

The process may be encountered during a normal or abnormal pregnancy, in association with trophoblastic disease or after ovulation induction. If the process follows ovulation induction, there may be multiple corpora lutea in addition to the follicle cysts.

14.5   Corpus luteum cyst

A cystic enlargement of the corpus luteum over 3 cm in diameter.

14.6   Pregnancy luteoma (Fig. 144)

Single or multiple nodules of lutein cells with abundant eosinophilic cytoplasm (Fig. 144) usually developing during an otherwise normal pregnancy.

These nodules are usually discovered incidentally when a caesarean section or a tubal ligation is being performed. They may attain a diameter of 15 cm or more. Mitotic figures may be numerous. Pregnancy luteomas are not autonomous tumours, but depend on hCG stimulation during pregnancy for their structural and functional integrity. Occasionally, they are virilizing. In a few cases, microscopic examination has disclosed postpartum degeneration of the nodules.

The pregnancy luteoma should be distinguished from the corpus luteum of pregnancy and steroid cell tumours. The corpus luteum of pregnancy has a festooned margin and contains both granulosa and theca lutein cells; colloid droplets and small foci of calcification are typically present. An association with pregnancy, multiplicity, mitotic activity and an absence or paucity of cytoplasmic lipid are helpful clues in differentiating the pregnancy luteoma from a steroid cell tumour, but such a distinction may be impossible in cases in which only a solitary lipid-free mass is present.

14.7   Ectopic pregnancy

This very rare occurrence may result in a haemorrhagic ovarian mass containing trophoblast and simulating a choriocarcinoma.

14.8   Stromal hyperplasia

A bilateral, occasionally tumour-like ovarian enlargement composed of proliferating ovarian stroma, which may be nodular or diffuse and may replace a portion of the ovary or the entire organ.

The exclusive or predominant cell type is a spindle cell that is smaller than that of a fibroma or fibromatosis and produces little collagen.

14.9   Stromal hyperthecosis (Figs. 145, 146)

A bilateral, occasionally tumour-like ovarian enlargement composed of proliferating ovarian stroma containing scattered clusters of lutein cells.

Stromal hyperthecosis is very rarely unilateral, whereas the luteinized thecoma is almost always unilateral. Stromal hyperthecosis may be associated with endocrine manifestations, which are usually androgenic, but occasionally oestrogenic.

14.10   Massive oedema (Fig. 147)

Marked enlargement of one or both ovaries by a stromal accumulation of oedema fluid that surrounds normal follicular structures.

In contrast, oedematous fibromas typically destroy or displace rather than envelop normal follicular structures.

In some cases of massive oedema, the stroma contains lutein cells and the patient is virilized or sexually precocious.

14.11   Fibromatosis (Fig. 148)

Moderate to marked enlargement of one or both ovaries by a fibromatous proliferation of the stroma, which surrounds normal follicular structures, unlike a fibroma.

In some cases, the stroma contains lutein cells and the patient is virilized. Occasionally, small aggregates of sex cord-type cells are present in the proliferating stroma.

14.12   Endometriosis (Figs. 149, 150)

A process in which glands and stroma resembling endometrial glands and stroma are located outside the endomyometrium (Figs. 149); rarely, only stroma is present in the form of small nodules in the outer ovarian cortex.

The stroma may be scanty or absent in postmenopausal women. Endometriosis may result in the formation of a large "chocolate" cyst simulating an ovarian cystic tumour. Hyperplasia of various types (Fig. 150) and a wide variety of tumours similar to those originating in the endometrium may also arise in endometriosis.

14.13   Cyst, unclassified (simple cyst)

A cyst without an identifiable lining.

Some cysts of this type may be cystadenomas and others follicle cysts, the linings of which have been destroyed.

14.14   Inflammatory lesions

These include, among others, inflammatory pseudotumour, xanthogranuloma, malakoplakia, infections, which are usually associated with salpingitis or intestinal disease, and echinococcal cysts.

TNM Classification of Tumours of the Ovary[1]

The definitions of the T, N and M categories correspond to the FIGO stages. both systems are included for comparison.

Rules for Classification

There should be histological confirmation of the disease and division of cases by histological type. The degree of differentiation (grade) should be recorded.

The following are the procedures for assessing T, N and M categories:

T categories	Physical examination, imaging, laparoscopy and/or surgical exploration
N categories	Physical examination, imaging, laparoscopy and/or surgical exploration
M categories	Physical examination, imaging, laparoscopy and/or surgical exploration

Regional Lymph Nodes

The regional lymph nodes are the hypogastric (obturator), common iliac, external iliac, lateral sacral, para-aortic and inguinal nodes.

---

[1] Sobin LH, Wittekind Ch (eds) (1997) TNM classification of malignant tumours, 5th edition. Wiley, New York. The figures on pp. 49-53 are reproduced from Hermanek P, Hutter RVP, Sobin LH, Wagner G, Wittekind Ch (eds) (1997) TNM Atlas, 4th edition. Springer, Berlin Heidelber New York.

TNM Clinical Classification

T – Primary Tumour

TNM Categories	FIGO Stages	
TX		Primary tumour cannot be assessed
T0		No evidence of primary tumour
T1	I	Tumour limited to the ovaries
T1a	IA	Tumour limited to one ovary; capsule intact, no tumour on ovarian surface; no malignant cells in ascites or peritoneal washings
T1b	IB	Tumour limited to both ovaries; capsule intact, no tumour on ovarian surface; no malignant cells in ascites or peritoneal washings
T1c	IC	Tumour limited to one or both ovaries with any of the following: capsule ruptured, tumour on ovarian surface, malignant cells in ascites or peritoneal washings
T2	II	Tumour involves one or both ovaries with pelvic extension
T2a	IIA	Extension and/or implants on uterus and/or tube(s); no malignant cells in ascites or peritoneal washings
T2b	IIB	Extension to other pelvic tissues; no malignant cells in ascites or peritoneal washings
T2c	IIC	Pelvic extension (2a or 2b) with malignant cells in ascites or peritoneal washings
T3 and/or N1	III	Tumour involves one or both ovaries with microscopically confirmed peritoneal metastasis outside the pelvis and/or regional lymph node metastasis
T3a	IIA	Microscopic peritoneal metastasis beyond pelvis
T3b	IIIB	Macroscopic peritoneal metastasis beyond pelvis 2 cm or less in greatest dimension

TNM Categories	*FIGO Stages*	
T3c and/or N1	IIIC	Peritoneal metastasis beyond pelvis more than 2 cm in greatest dimension and/or regional lymph node metastasis
M1	IV	Distant metastasis (excludes peritoneal metastasis)

Note: Liver capsule metastasis is T3/stage II, liver parenchymal metastasis M1/stage IV. Pleural effusion must have positive cytology for M1/stage IV.

N – Regional Lymph Nodes

NX	Regional lymph nodes cannot be assessed
N0	No regional lymph node metastasis
N1	Regional lymph node metastasis

M – Distant Metastasis

MX	Distant metastasis cannot be assessed
M0	No distant metastasis
M1	Distant metastasis

pTNM Pathological Classification

The pT, pN and pM categories correspond to the T, N and M categories.

pN0	Histological examination of a pelvic lymphadenectomy specimen will ordinarily include ten or more lymph nodes.

G – Histopathological Grading

GX	Grade cannot be assessed
GB	Borderline malignancy
G1	Well differentiated
G2	Moderately differentiated
G3–4	Poorly differentiated or undifferentiated

Stage Grouping

Stage IA	T1a	N0	M0
Stage IB	T1b	N0	M0
Stage IC	T1c	N0	M0
Stage IIA	T2a	N0	M0
Stage IIB	T2b	N0	M0
Stage IIC	T2c	N0	M0
Stage IIIA	T3a	N0	M0
Stage IIIB	T3b	N0	M0
Stage IIIC	T3c	N0	M0
	Any T	N1	M0
Stage IV	Any T	Any N	M1

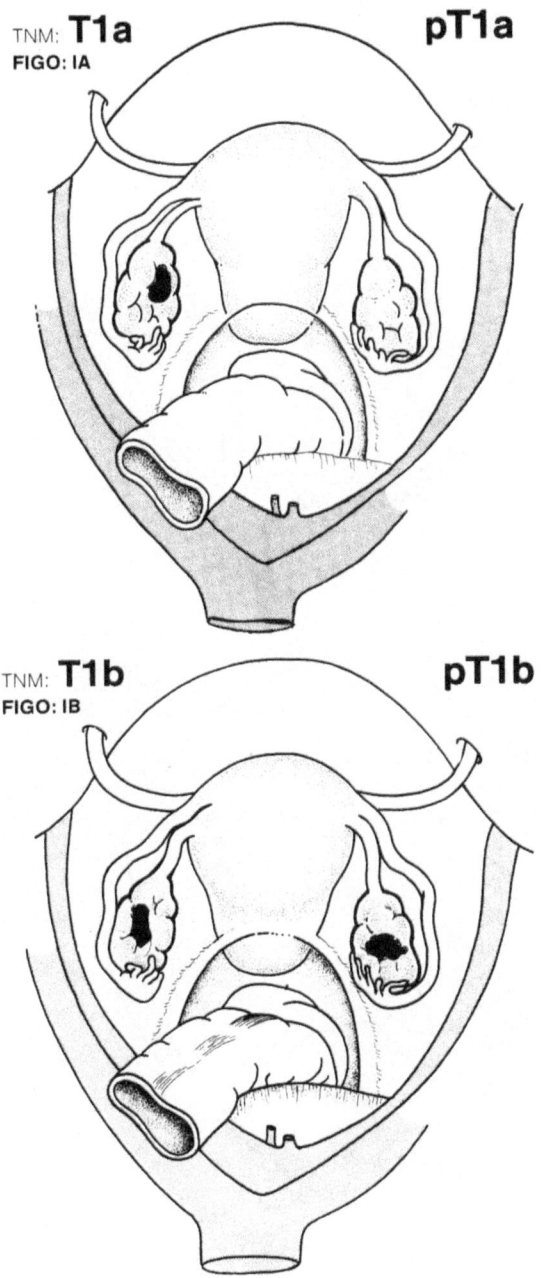

TNM: **T1a**
FIGO: IA

pT1a

TNM: **T1b**
FIGO: IB

pT1b

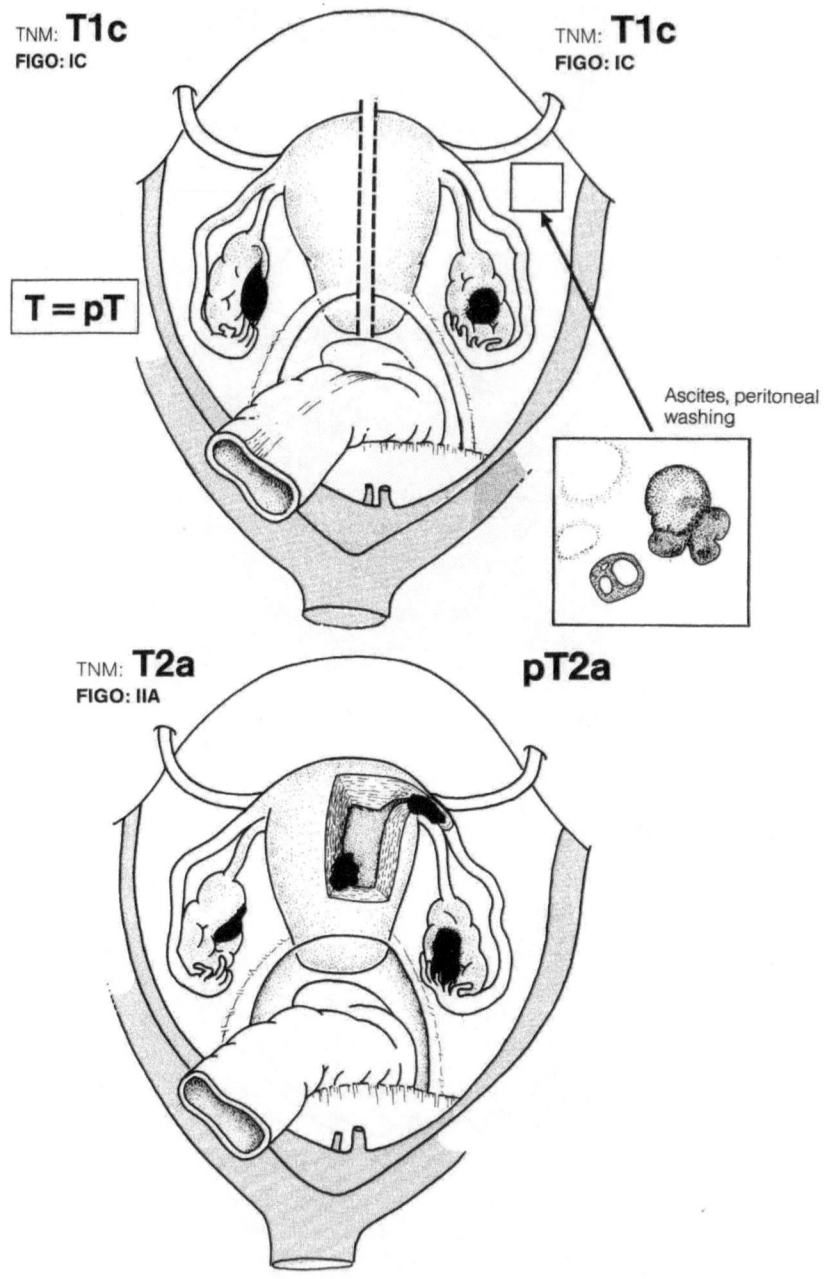

TNM: **T1c**
FIGO: IC

TNM: **T1c**
FIGO: IC

T = pT

Ascites, peritoneal washing

TNM: **T2a**
FIGO: IIA

pT2a

TNM: **T2b**
FIGO: IIB

pT2b

TNM: **T2c**
FIGO: IIC ›

pT2c

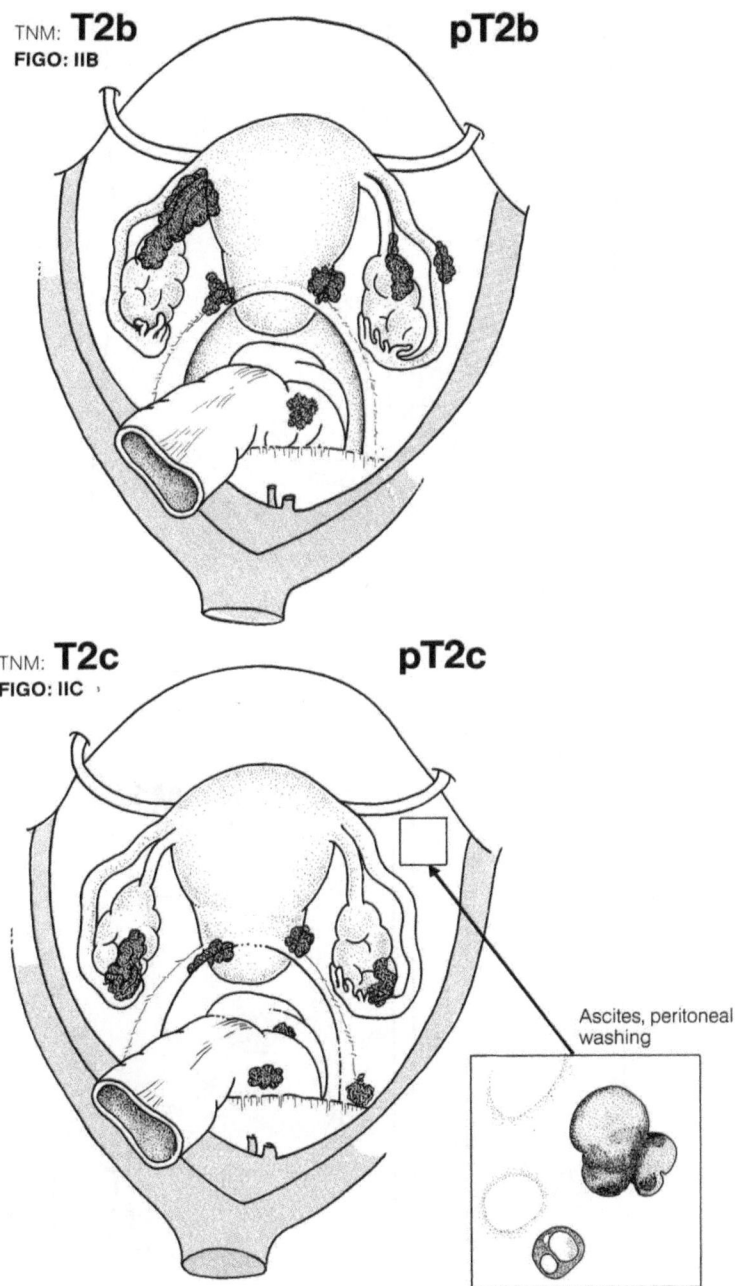

Ascites, peritoneal
washing

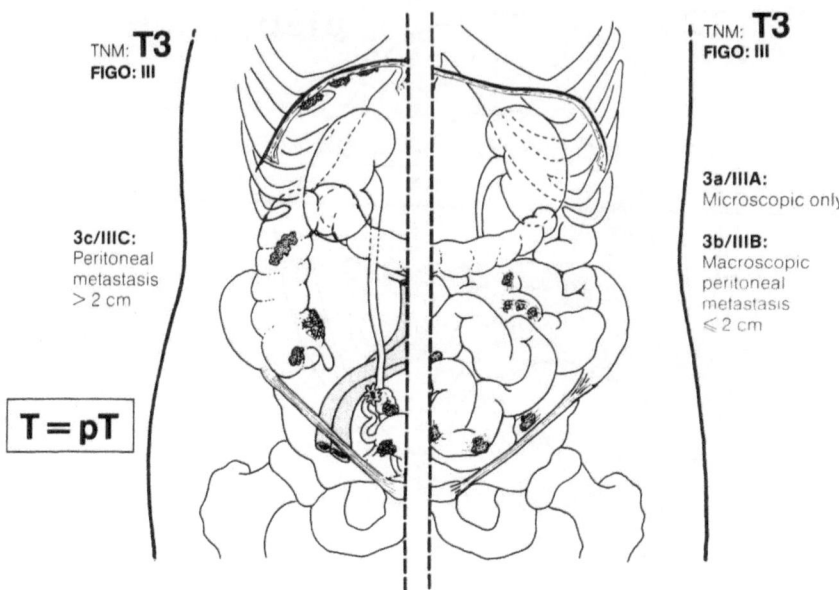

TNM: **T3**
FIGO: III

TNM: **T3**
FIGO: III

3a/IIIA:
Microscopic only

3b/IIIB:
Macroscopic
peritoneal
metastasis
≤ 2 cm

3c/IIIC:
Peritoneal
metastasis
> 2 cm

T = pT

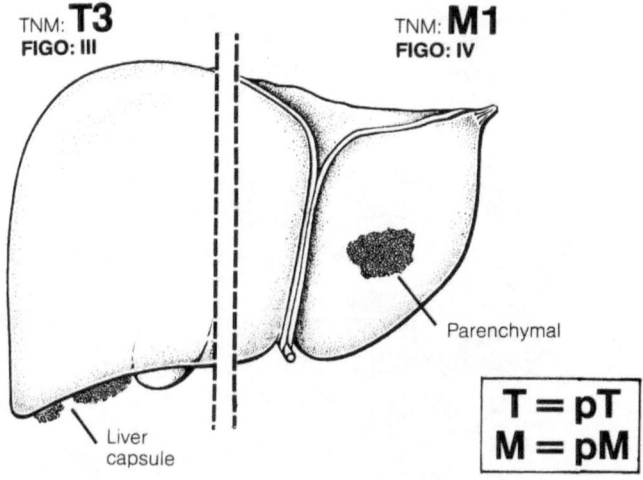

TNM: **T3**
FIGO: III

TNM: **M1**
FIGO: IV

Parenchymal

Liver
capsule

T = pT
M = pM

N1

pN1

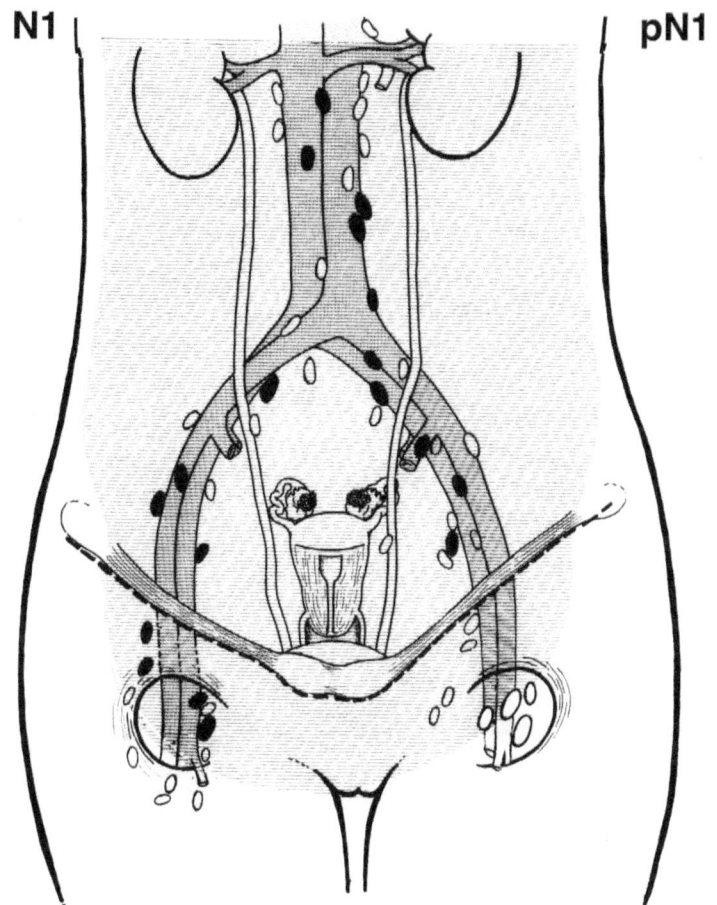

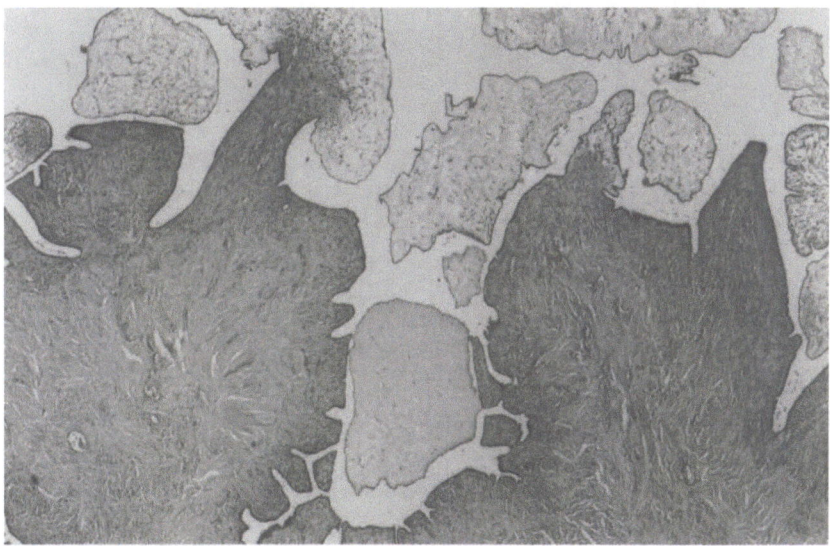

Fig. 1. *Serous papillary cystadenoma*. Oedematous and densely collagenous fibrous papillae lined by cuboidal and flat epithelial cells

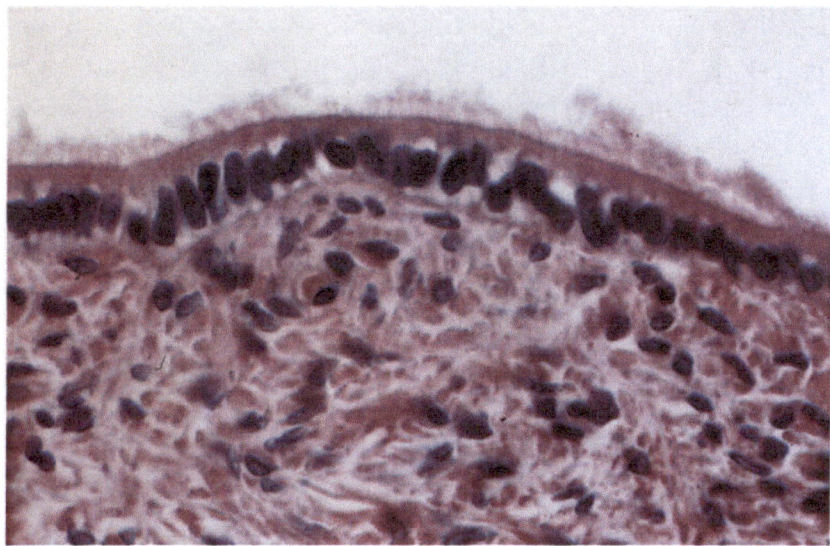

Fig. 2. *Serous cystadenoma*. Ciliated epithelium of cyst adjacent to stromal component

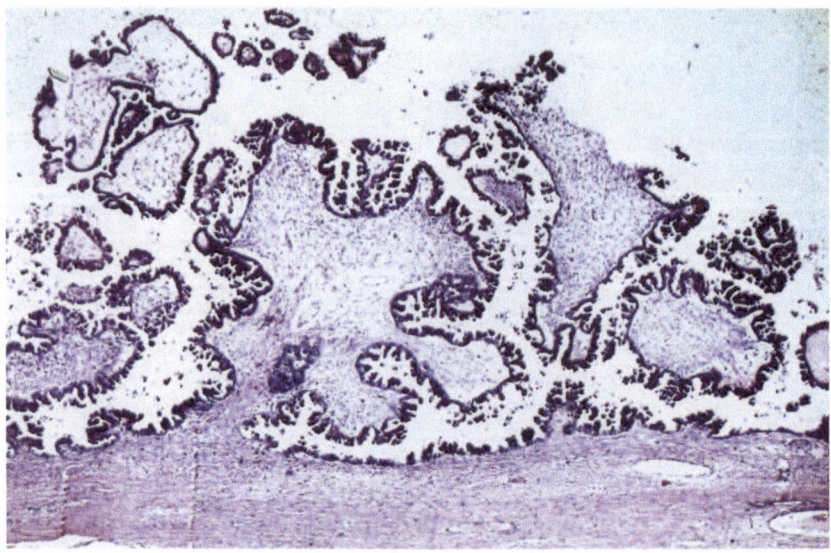

Fig. 3. *Serous papillary cystic tumour of borderline malignancy.* Stratification with cellular budding of epithelial cells and absence of invasion

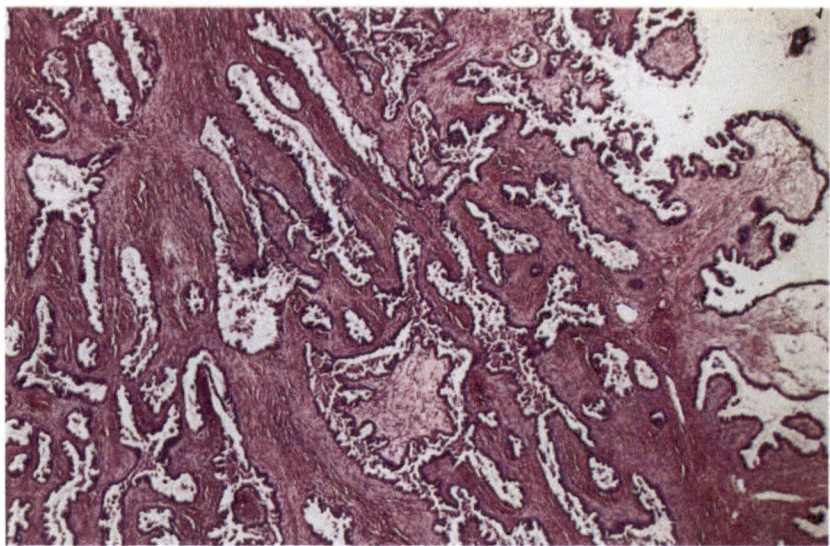

Fig. 4. *Serous papillary cystic tumour of borderline malignancy.* Orderly penetration of stromal component by epithelial units without stromal reaction

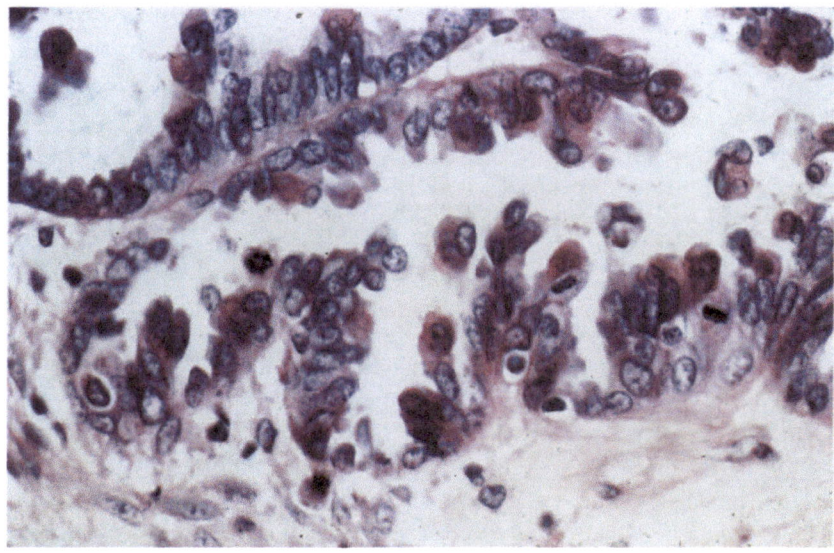

Fig. 5. *Serous papillary cystic tumour of borderline malignancy.* Moderate nuclear atypicality and mitotic activity

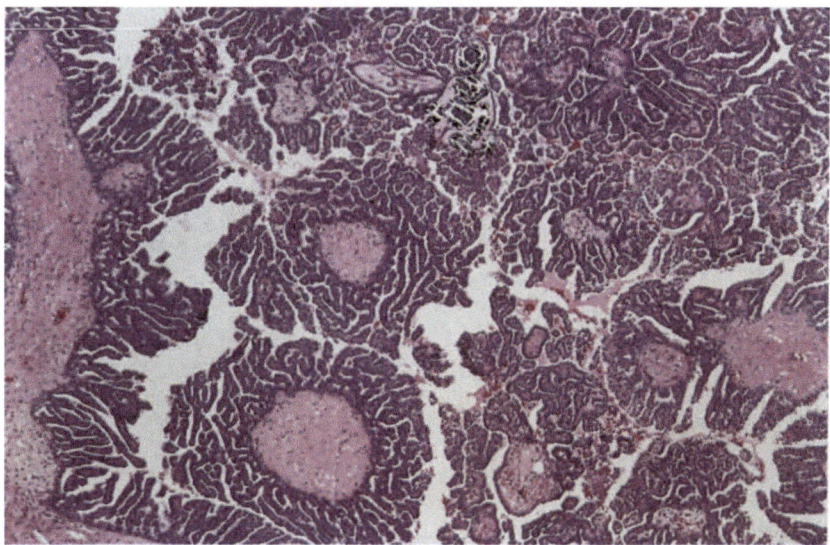

Fig. 6. *Serous papillary cystic tumour of borderline malignancy.* Micropapillary pattern

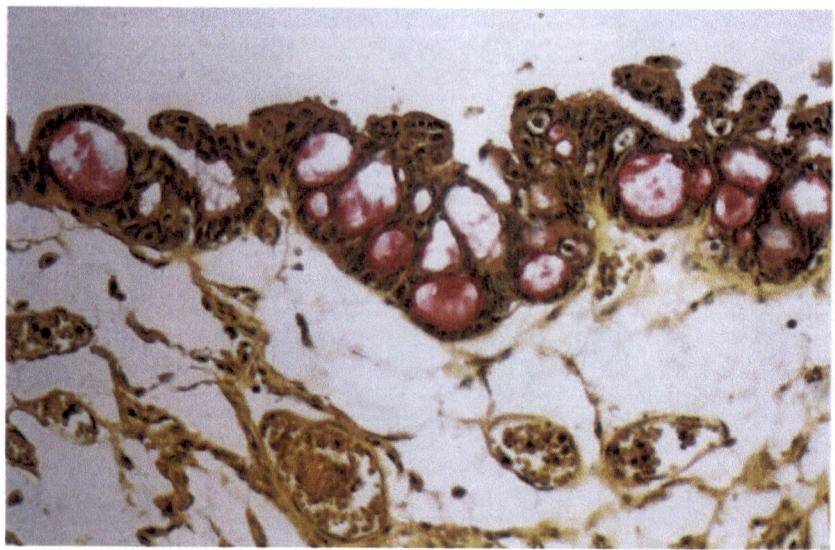

Fig. 7. *Serous papillary cystic tumour of borderline malignancy.* Cribriform pattern. Mucicarmine stain

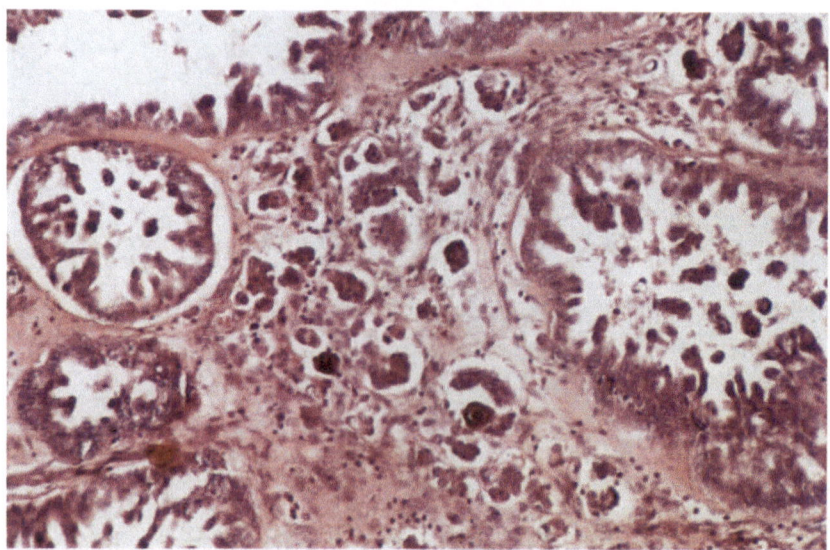

Fig. 8. *Serous papillary cystic tumour of borderline malignancy.* Microinvasion of stroma. [From Young RH, Clement PB, Scully RE (1994) The ovary. In: Sternberg SS (ed) Diagnostic surgical pathology. Raven, New York, pp 2195–2279]

59

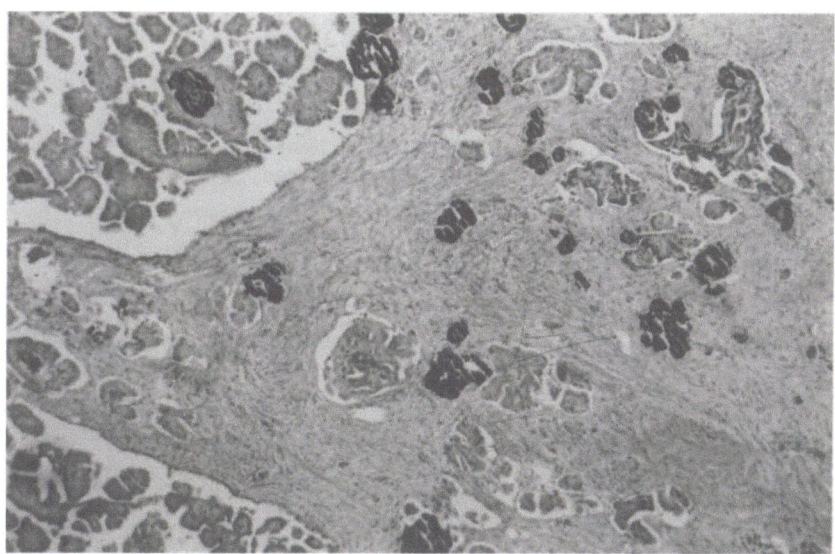

Fig. 9. *Serous papillary adenocarcinoma.* Obvious stromal invasion with desmoplastic stromal reaction and calcification of many epithelial nests. [From Scully RE (1968) Classification, pathology and biologic behavior of ovarian tumors. Nassau County Med Center Proc 1:148–163]

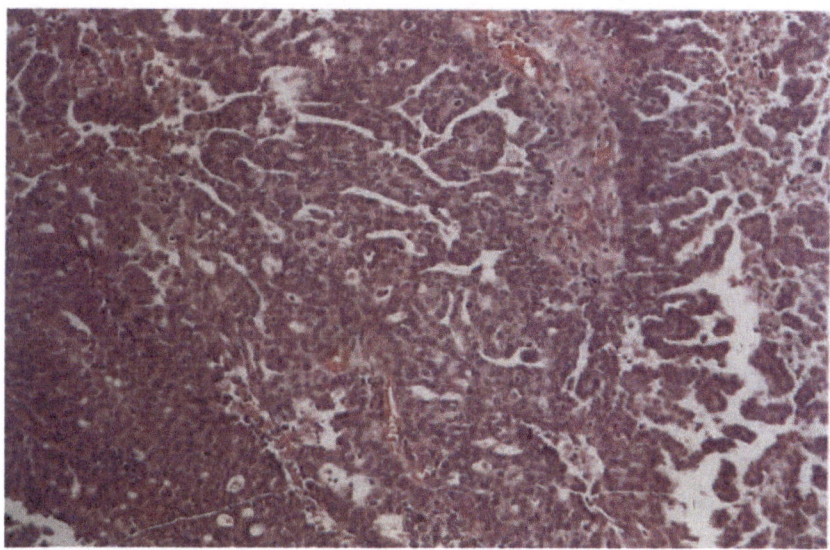

Fig. 10. *Serous papillary adenocarcinoma.* Irregular thin cellular papillae and slit-like lumens. [From Scully RE, Young RH, Clement PB (1998) Tumors of the ovary, maldeveloped gonads, fallopian tube, and broad ligament. Atlas of tumor pathology, 3rd series. Armed Forces Institute of Pathology, Washington, DC]

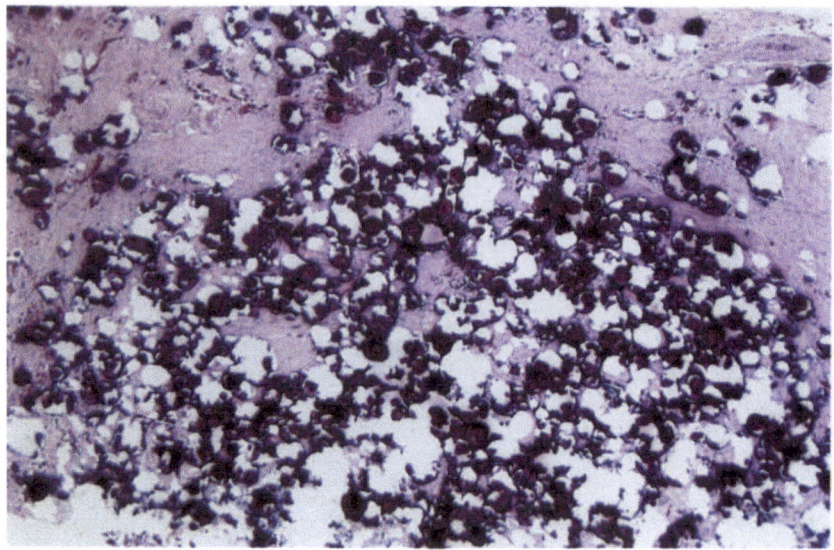

Fig. 11. *Serous papillary carcinoma.* Psammocarcinoma variant

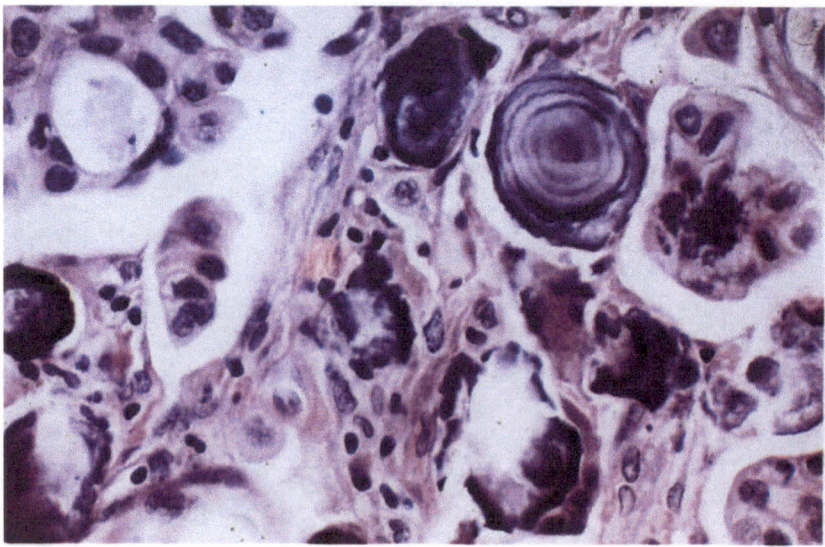

Fig. 12. *Serous papillary carcinoma.* Characteristic lamination of psammoma body

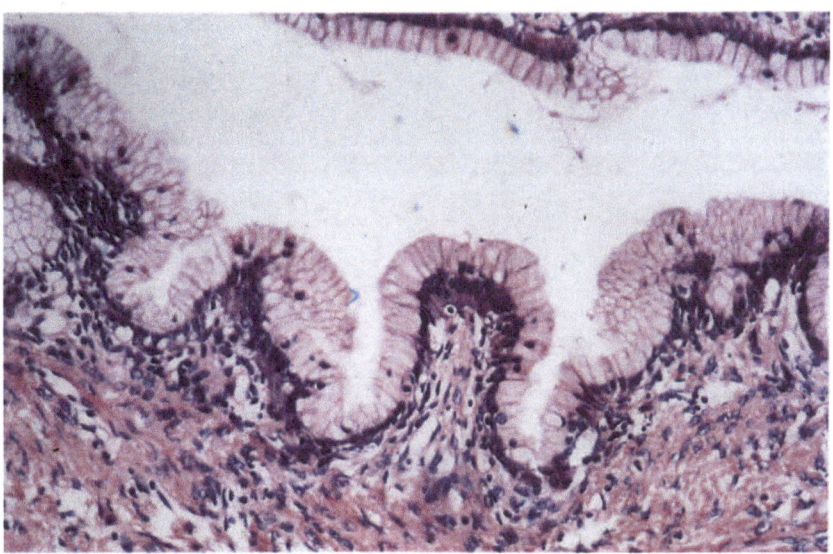

Fig. 13. *Mucinous cystadenoma*. Cyst lined by benign endocervical-like epithelium

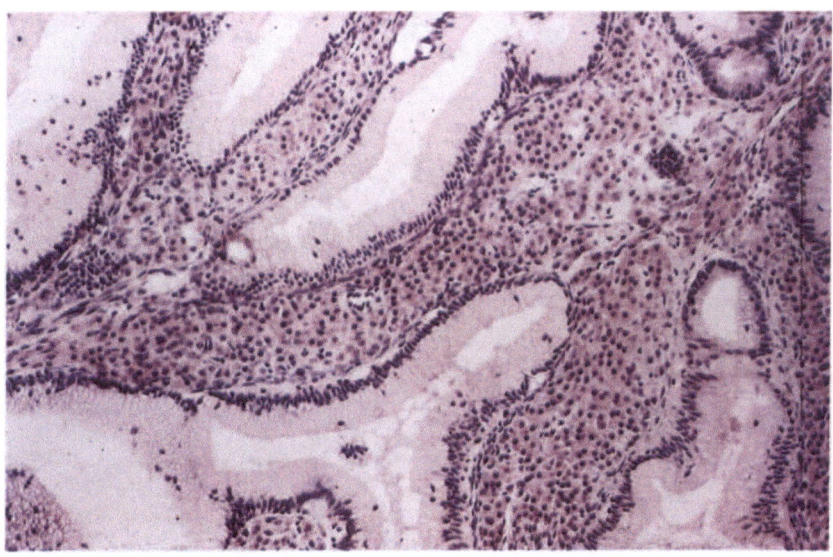

Fig. 14. *Mucinous cystadenoma*. Luteinization of stromal component in virilized pregnant patient

62

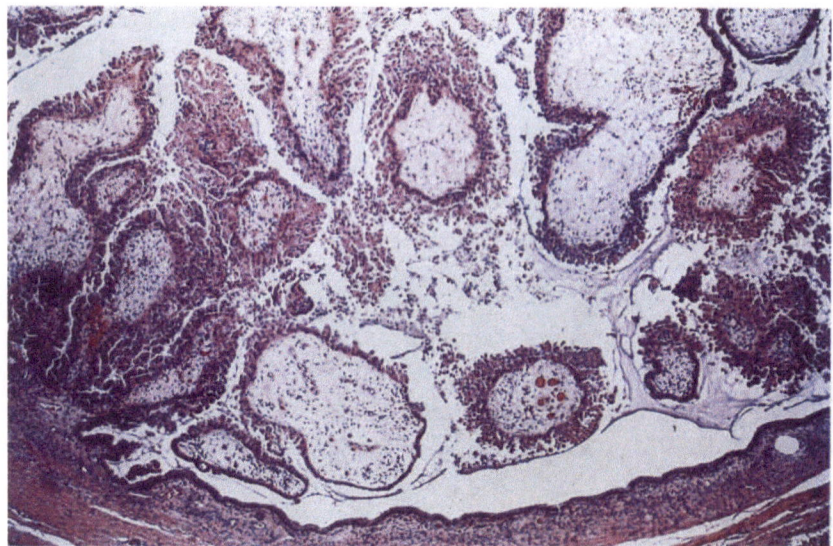

Fig. 15. *Mucinous papillary cystic tumour of borderline malignancy of endocervical-like type.* Stratified mucinous epithelium with cellular budding lining oedematous papillae

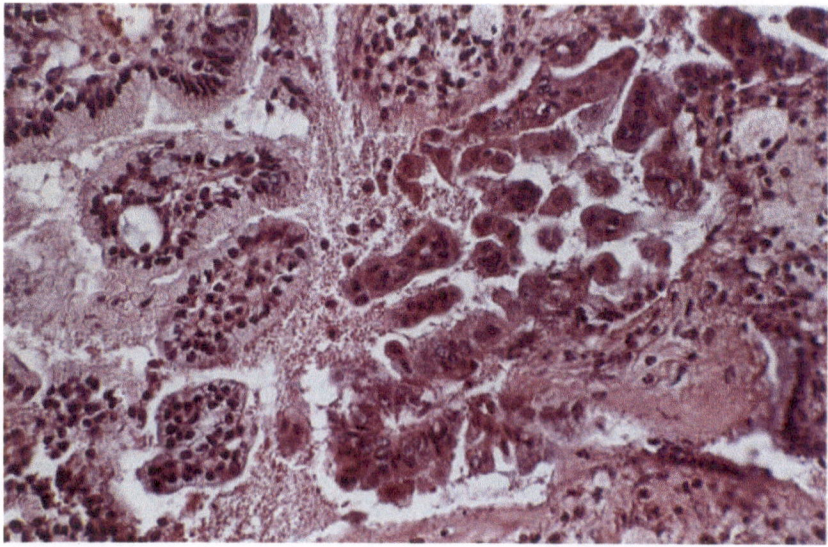

Fig. 16. *Mucinous papillary cystic tumour of borderline malignancy of endocervical-like type.* Epithelial cells filled with mucin and cellular budding

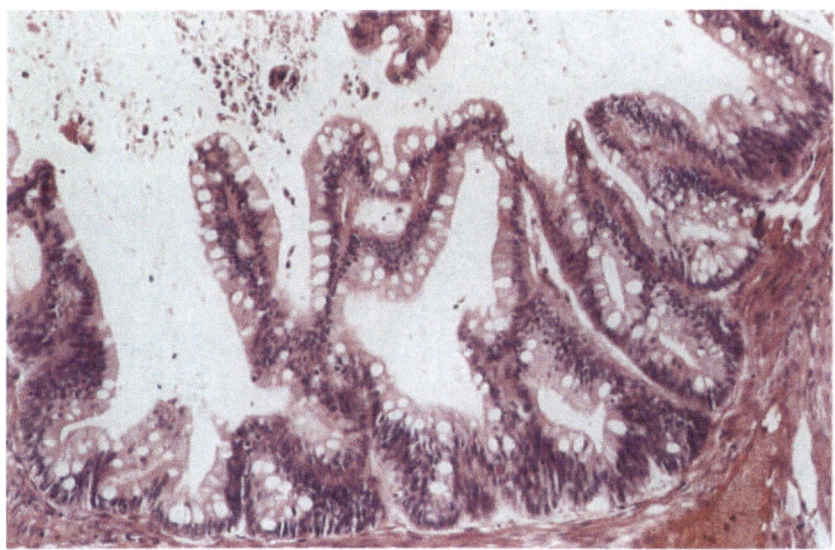

Fig. 17. *Mucinous papillary cystic tumour of borderline malignancy of intestinal type.* Branching filiform papillae lined by mucinous epithelium containing goblet cells

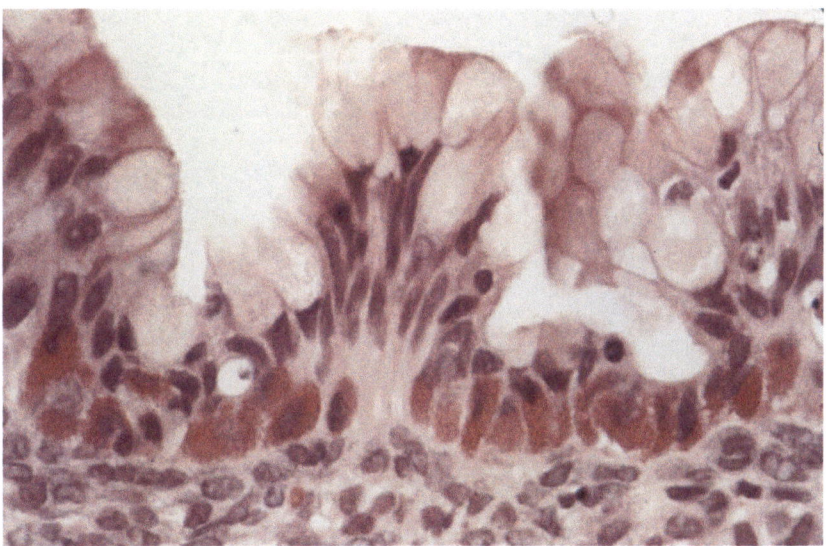

Fig. 18. *Mucinous papillary cystic tumour of borderline malignancy of intestinal type.* Argentaffin cells with orange granules in cytoplasm and goblet cells. [From Scully RE, Young RH, Clement PB (1998) Tumors of the ovary, maldeveloped gonads, fallopian tube, and broad ligament. Atlas of tumor pathology, 3rd series. Armed Forces Institute of Pathology, Washington, DC]

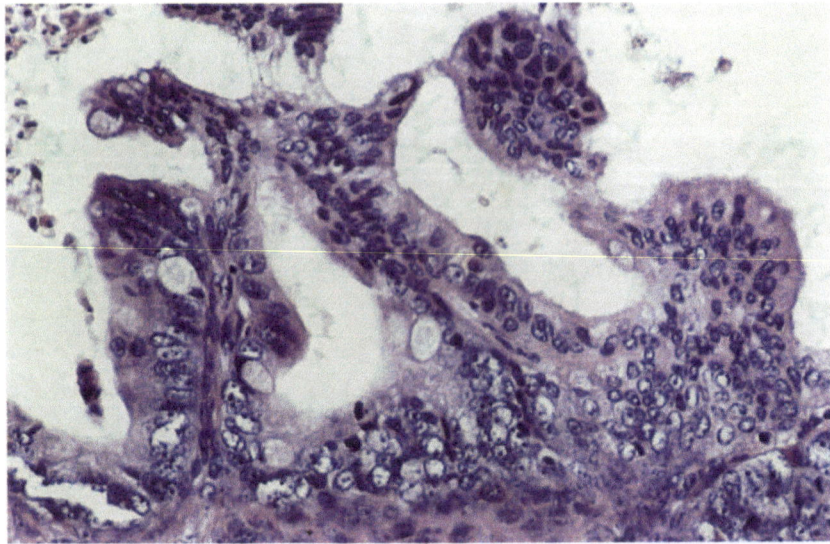

Fig. 19. *Mucinous cystic tumour of borderline malignancy of intestinal type.* Intra-epithelial carcinoma characterized by marked nuclear atypicality and mitotic activity

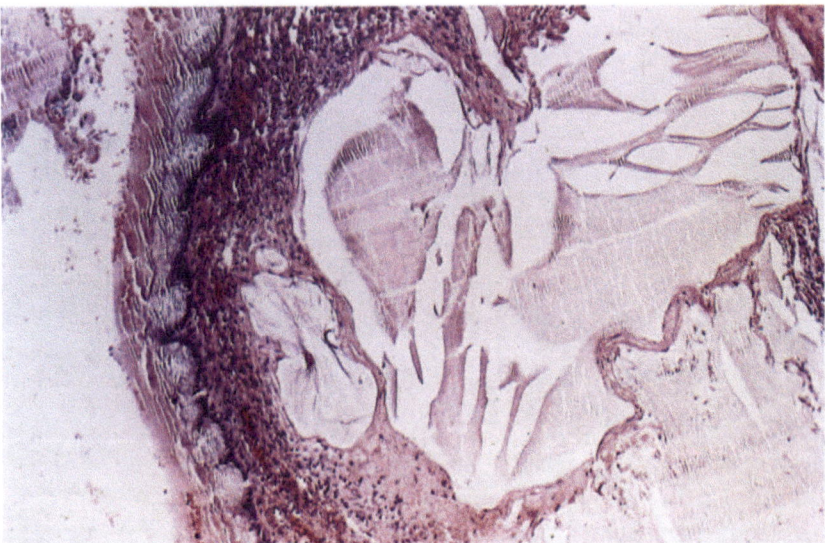

Fig. 20. *Mucinous cystic tumour associated with pseudomyxoma peritonei.* High-co-lumnar mucinous epithelium and stromal pools of mucin (pseudomyxoma ovarii)

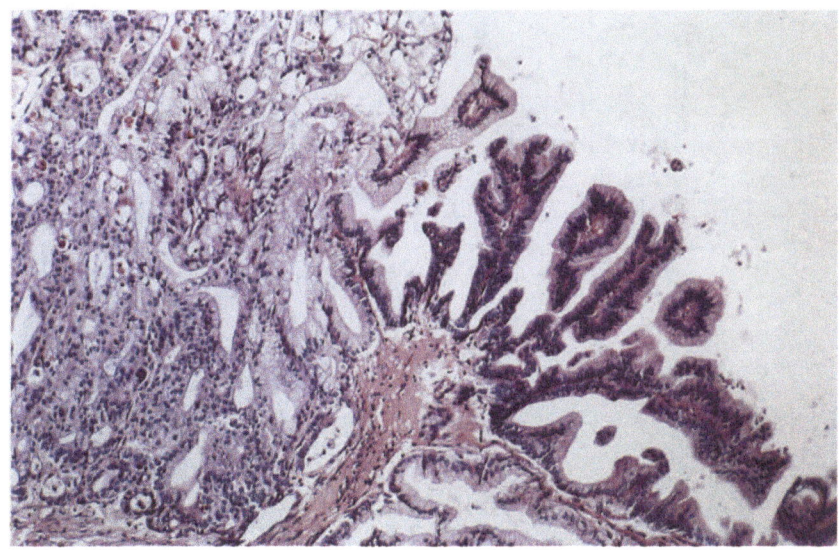

Fig. 21. *Mucinous adenocarcinoma (left) and mucinous papillary cystic tumour of borderline malignancy of intestinal type (right).* Expansile type of stromal invasion with back-to-back glands

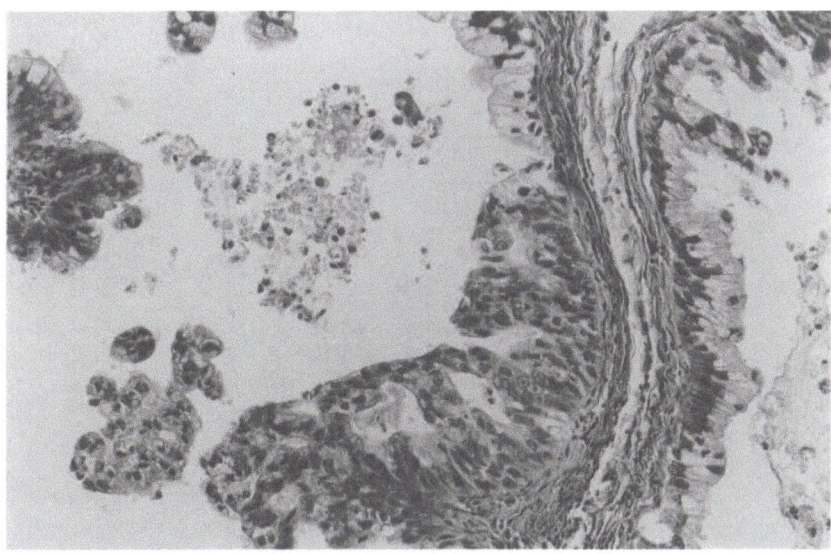

Fig. 22. *Mucinous adenocarcinoma.* Cysts lined by mucinous epithelium, with marked stratification and nuclear atypicality in larger cyst with "dirty" necrotic material in lumen

66

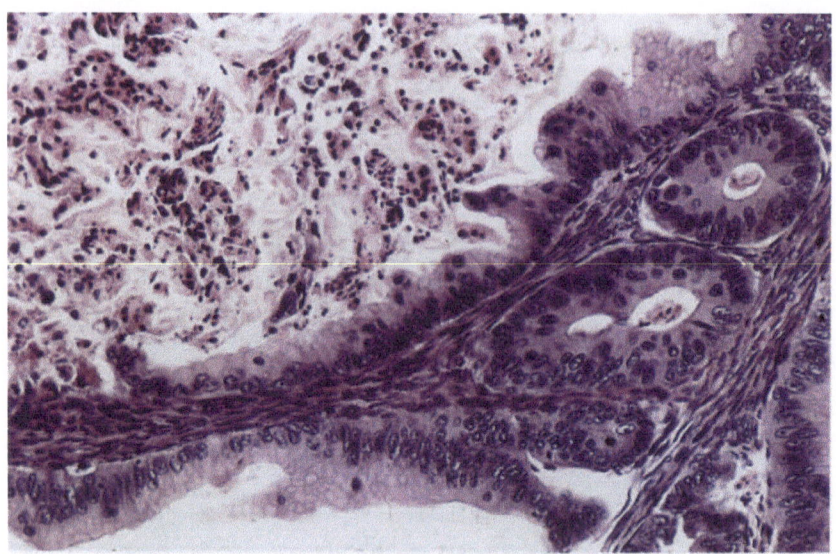

Fig. 23. *Mucinous adenocarcinoma.* Mucinous glands and cysts lined by mucinous and mucin-free cells and large cyst filled with "dirty" necrotic material

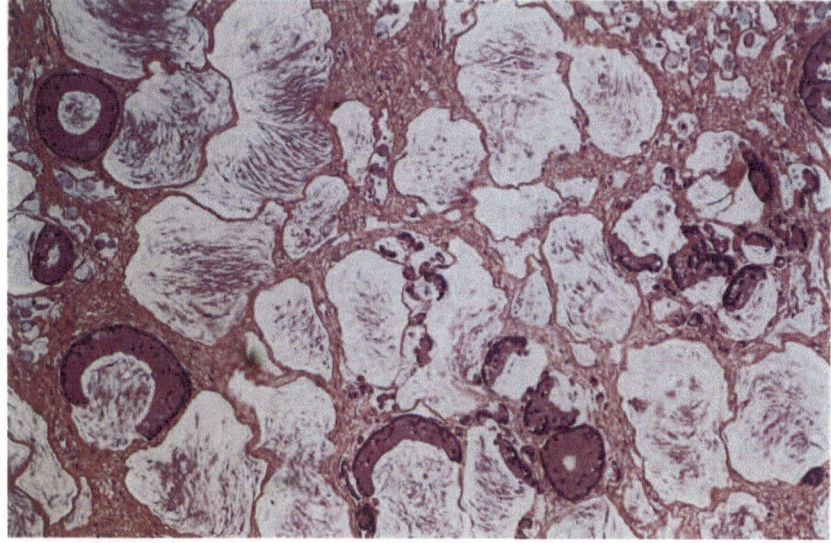

Fig. 24. *Mucinous adenocarcinoma.* Resemblance to "colloid" carcinoma of intestine

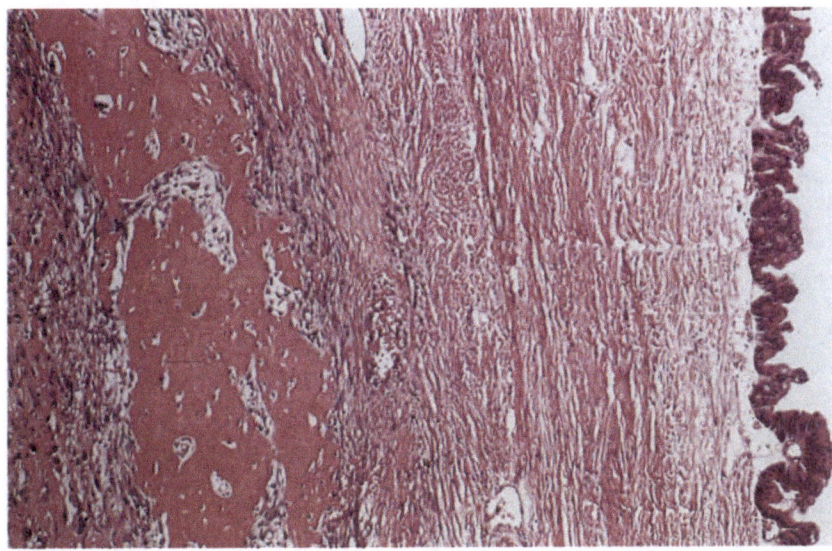

Fig. 25. *Mucinous cystic tumour of borderline malignancy of intestinal type.* Well-demarcated solid sarcoma-like nodule containing a bony trabeculum in cyst wall

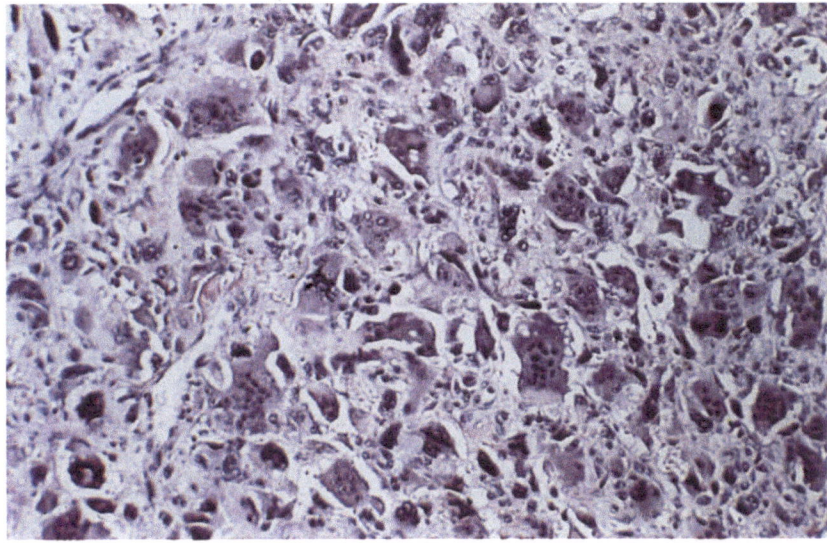

Fig. 26. *Sarcoma-like nodule in woll of mucinous cystic tumour.* Closely packed epulis-like giant cells, one of which has an atypical mitotic figure

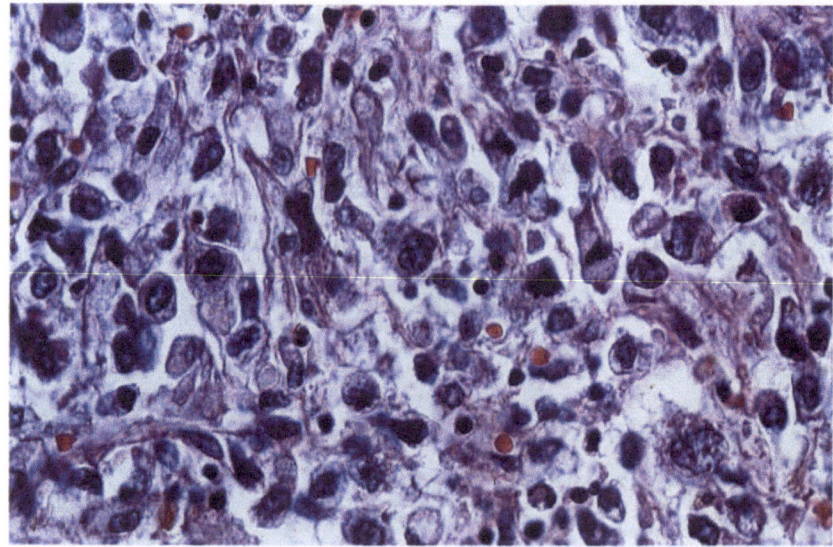

Fig. 27. *Anaplastic-carcinoma nodule in wall of mucinous cystic tumour.* Hyperchromatic nuclei and eosinophilic cytoplasm

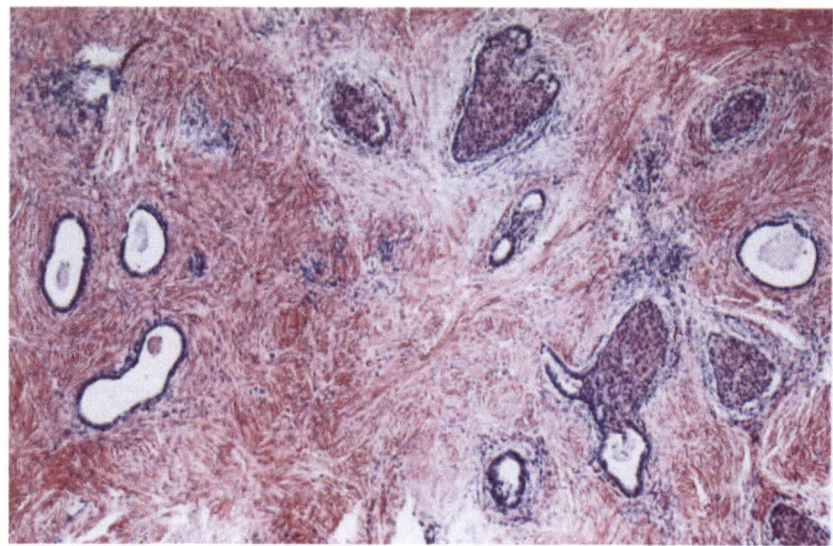

Fig. 28. *Endometrioid adenofibroma with squamous differentiation.* Squamous morules occupying some glands with surrounding fibrous stromal reaction

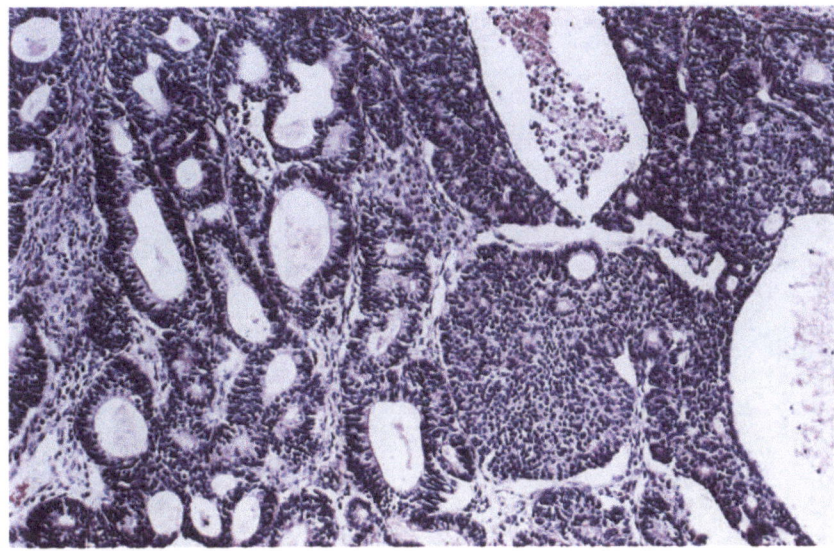

Fig. 29. *Endometrioid adenocarcinoma.* Tubular glands lined by stratified non-mucin-containing epithelium and solid areas of carcinoma

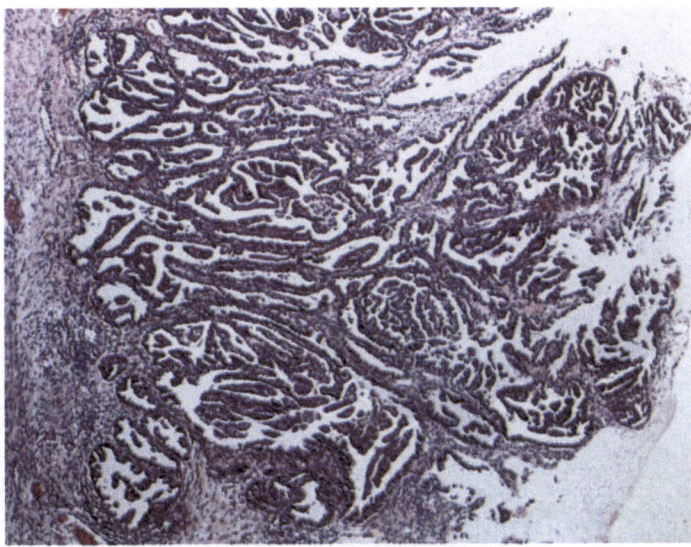

Fig. 30. *Endometrioid adenocarcinoma.* Villoglandular pattern of lining of cyst wall. [From Scully RE, Young RH, Clement PB (1998) Tumors of the ovary, maldeveloped gonads, fallopian tube, and broad ligament. Atlas of tumor pathology, 3rd series. Armed Forces Institute of Pathology, Washington, DC]

70

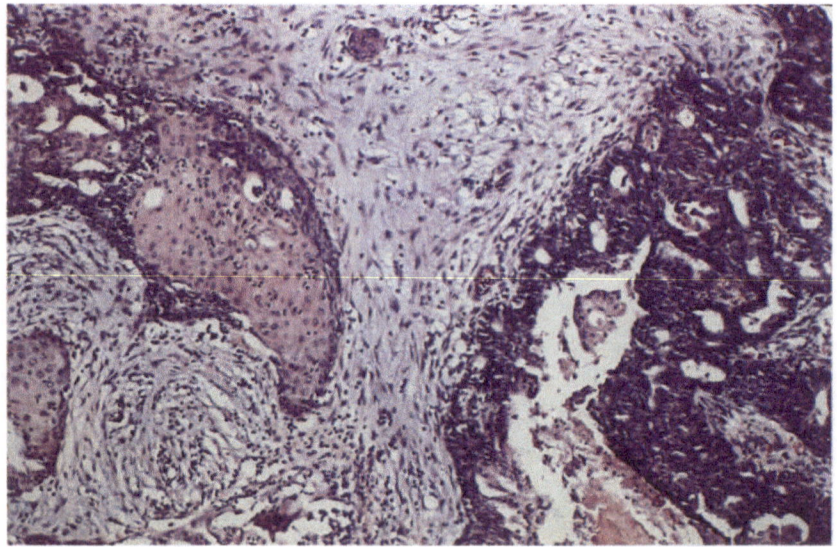

Fig. 31. *Endometrioid adenocarcinoma with squamous differentiation.* Conspicuous tooth-shaped squamous nest infiltrating stroma

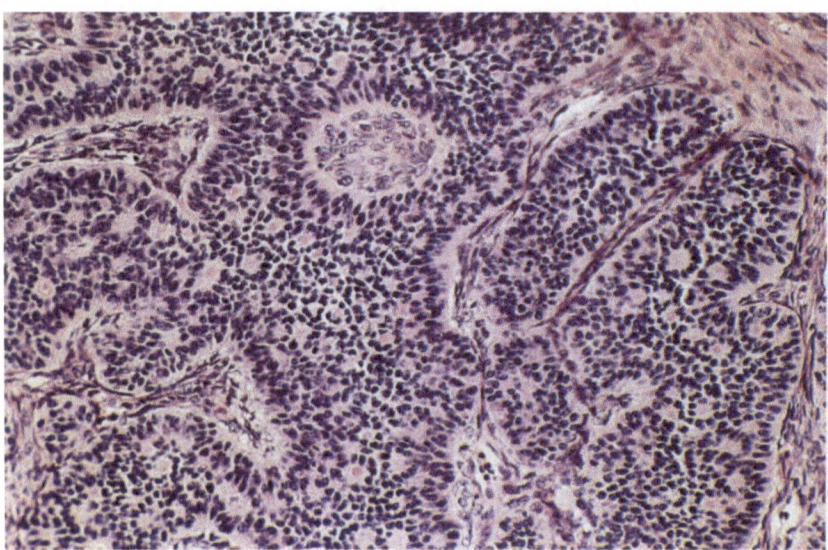

Fig. 32. *Endometrioid adenocarcinoma.* Architecture and microglandular pattern simulating microfollicular granulosa cell tumour. [From Scully RE, Young RH, Clement PB (1998) Tumors of the ovary, maldeveloped gonads, fallopian tube, and broad ligament. Atlas of tumor pathology, 3rd series. Armed Forces Institute of Pathology, Washington, DC]

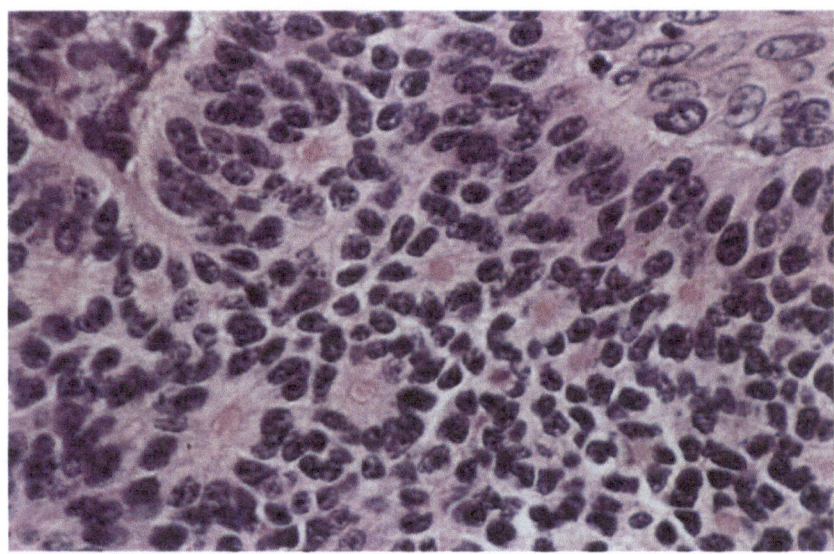

Fig. 33. *Endometrioid adenocarcinoma*. Microglandular pattern simulating microfollicular granulosa cell tumour but lacking pale nuclei of latter. [From Scully RE, Young RH, Clement PB (1998) Tumors of the ovary, maldeveloped gonads, fallopian tube, and broad ligament. Atlas of tumor pathology, 3rd series. Armed Forces Institute of Pathology, Washington, DC]

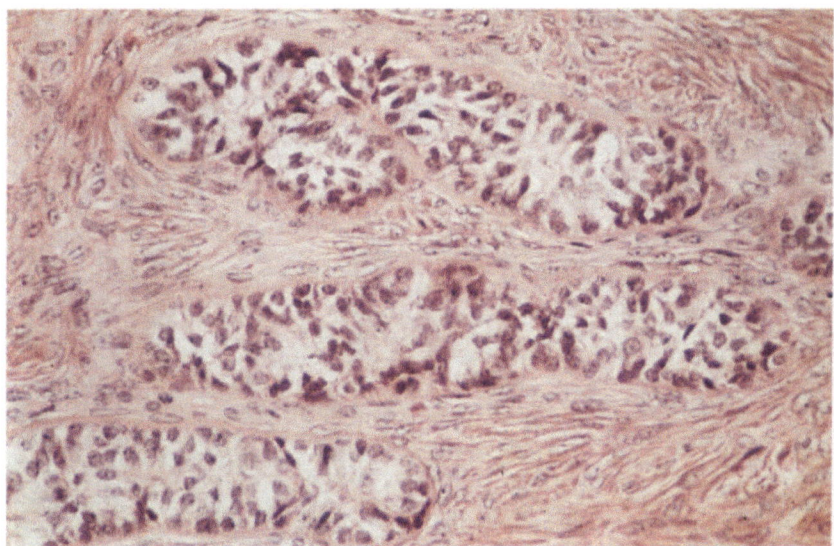

Fig. 34. *Endometrioid adenocarcinoma*. Solid tubules closely resembling those of Sertoli cell tumour

72

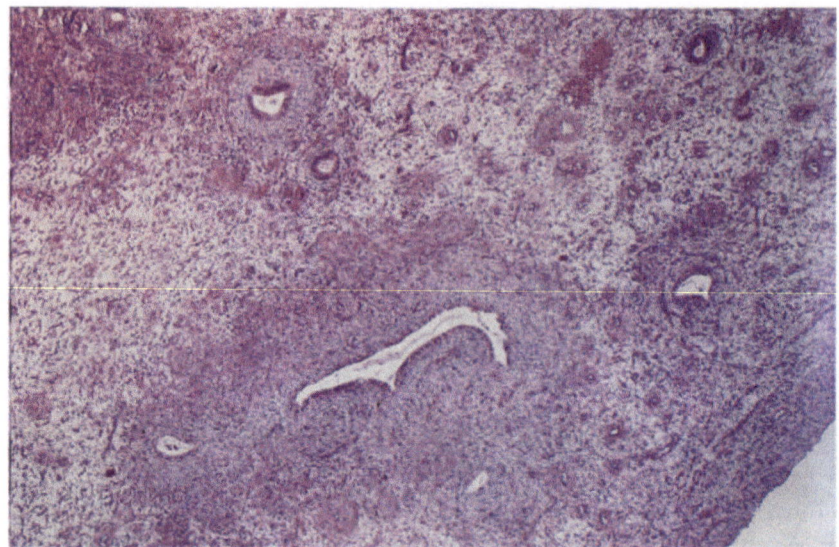

Fig. 35. *Endometrioid adenosarcoma.* Endometrioid glands surrounded by cuffs of cellular stromal component

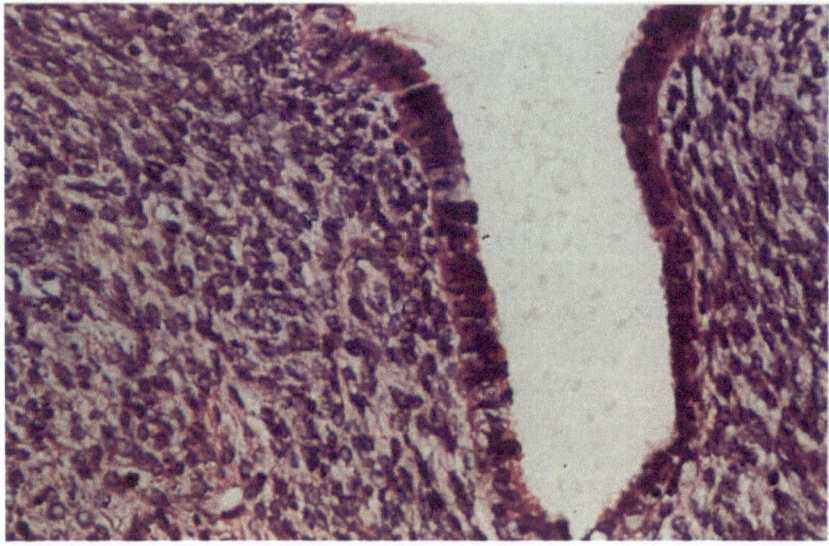

Fig. 36. *Endometrioid adenosarcoma.* Endometrioid glands and adjacent highly cellular stroma

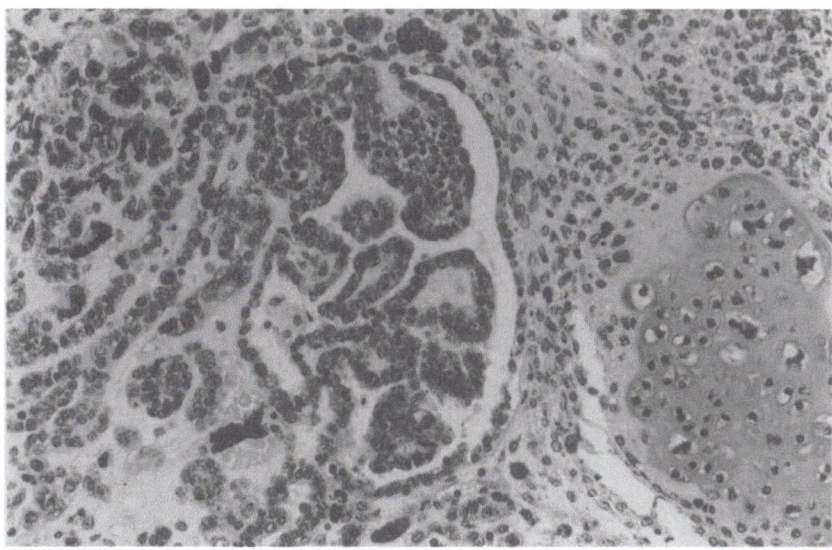

Fig. 37. *Malignant mesodermal mixed tumour.* Serous papillary carcinoma and island of cartilage containing atypical nuclei

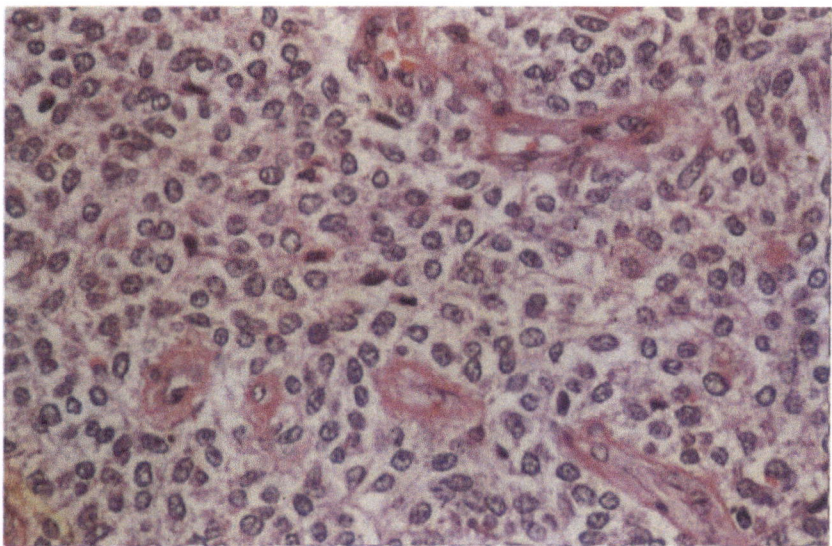

Fig. 38. *Endometrioid stromal sarcoma.* Diffuse arrangement of cells with pale nuclei and numerous arterioles. [From Scully RE, Young RH, Clement PB (1998) Tumors of the ovary, maldeveloped gonads, fallopian tube, and broad ligament. Atlas of tumor pathology, 3rd series. Armed Forces Institute of Pathology, Washington, DC]

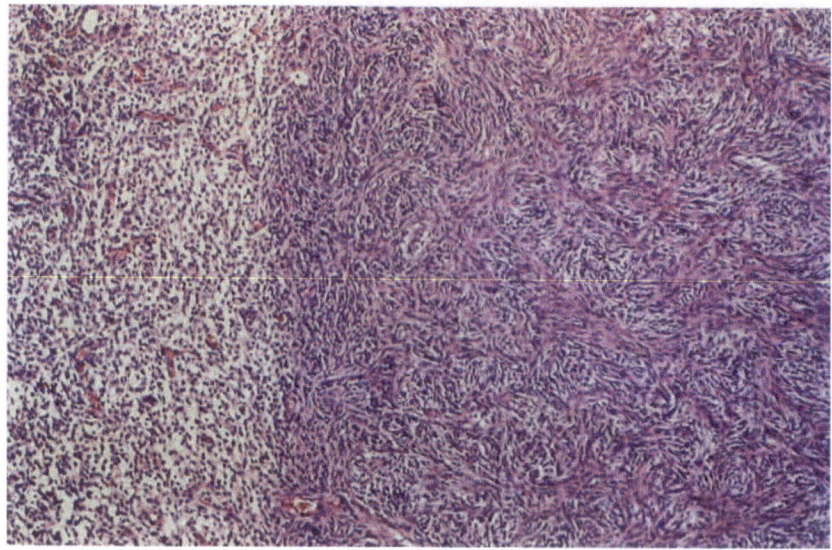

Fig. 39. *Endometrioid stromal sarcoma.* Pale typical component and darker fibromatous component. [From Scully RE, Young RH, Clement PB (1998) Tumors of the ovary, maldeveloped gonads, fallopian tube, and broad ligament. Atlas of tumor pathology, 3rd series. Armed Forces Institute of Pathology, Washington, DC]

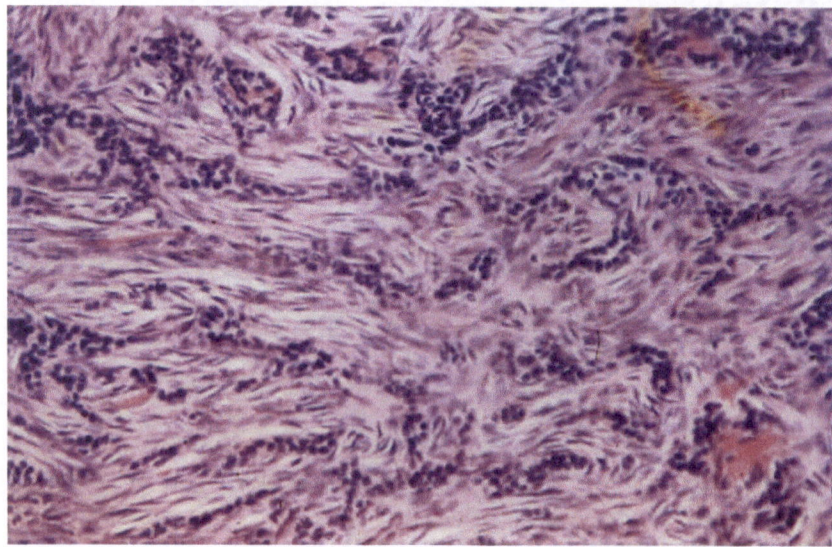

Fig. 40. *Endometrioid stromal sarcoma.* Sex cord-like differentiation in fibromatous component. [From Young RH, Clement PB, Scully RE (1994) The ovary. In: Sternberg SS (ed) Diagnostic surgical pathology. Raven, New York, pp 2195–2279]

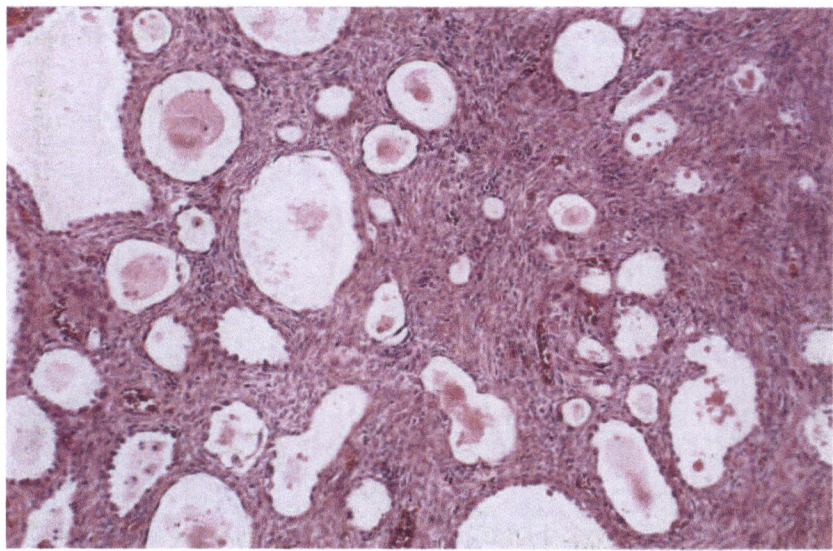

Fig. 41. *Clear cell adenofibroma of borderline malignancy.* Glands and small cysts lined by mostly flattened atypical hobnail cells without stromal invasion

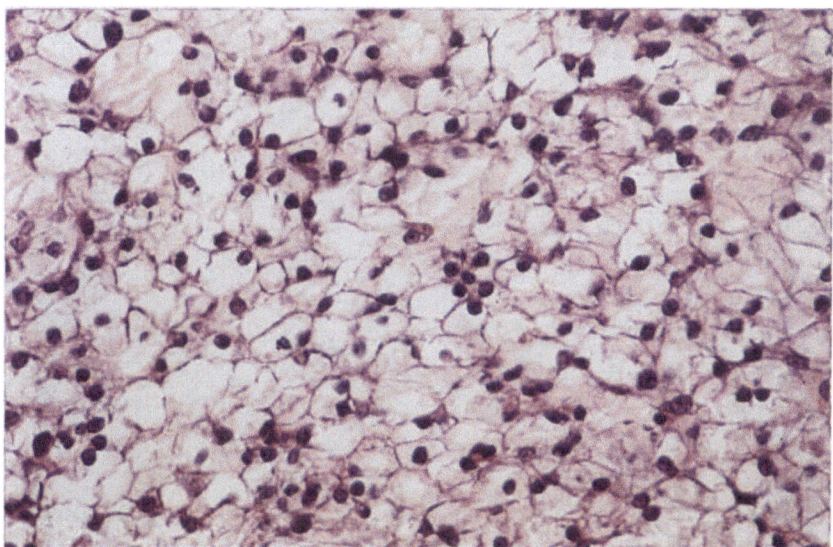

Fig. 42. *Clear cell carcinoma.* Diffuse arrangement of polyhedral clear cells with eccentric nuclei

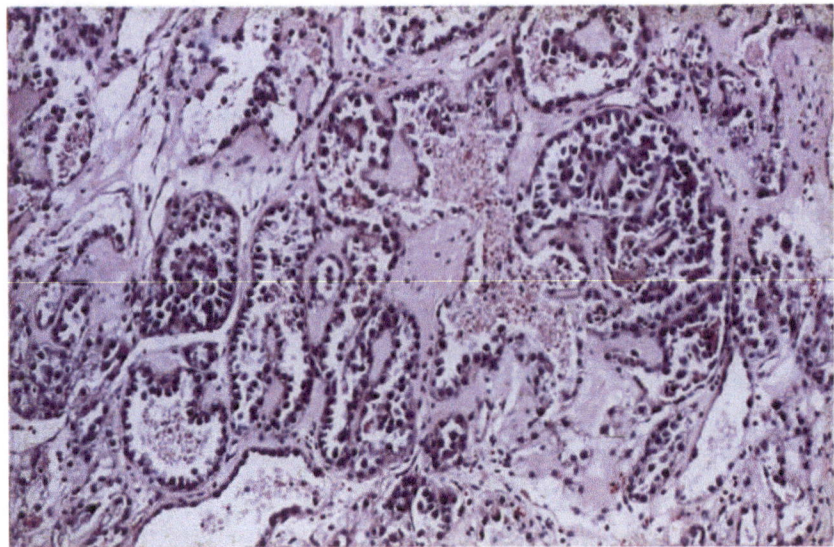

Fig. 43. *Clear cell papillary adenocarcinoma.* Tubules and their papillae lined by hobnail cells

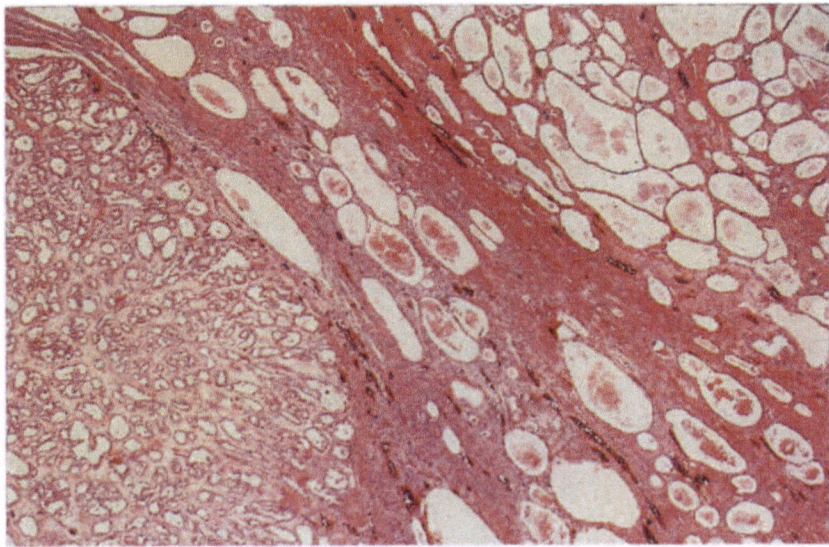

Fig. 44. *Clear cell adenocarcinoma.* Small glands and cystic glands lined by cuboidal and flat epithelium, respectively

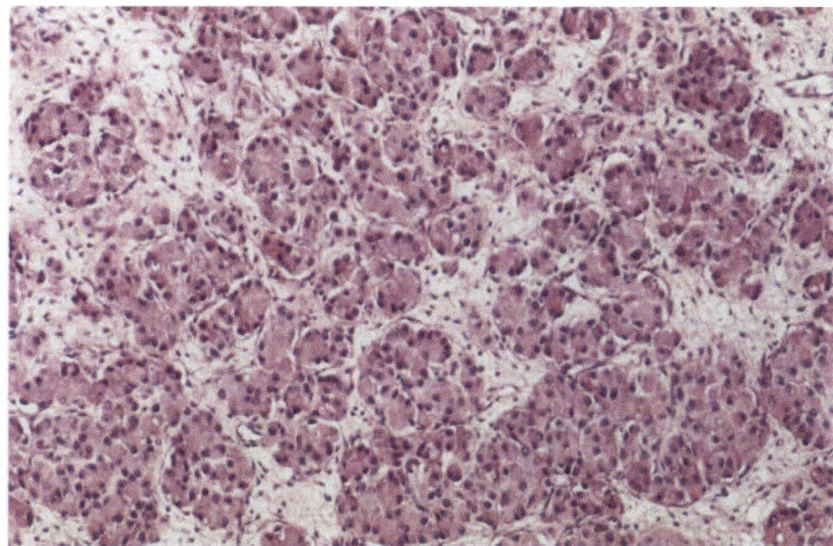

Fig. 45. *Clear cell carcinoma*. Nests and larger aggregates composed of oxyphil cells

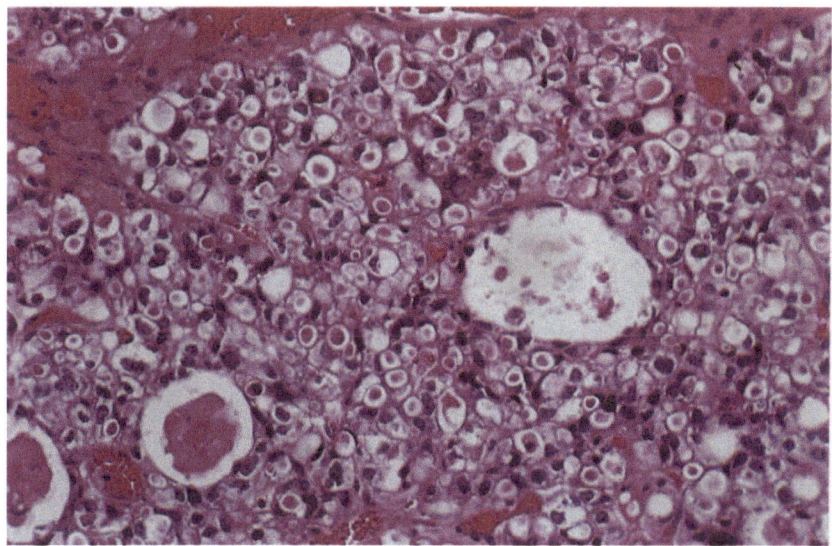

Fig. 46. *Clear cell adenocarcinoma*. Cells filled with mucin with a bull's-eye distribution

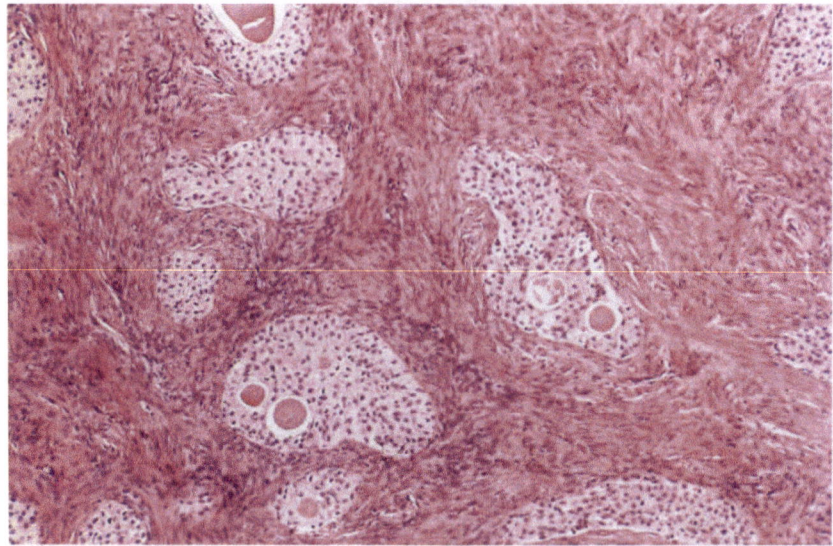

Fig. 47. *Brenner tumour.* Rounded solid nests of transitional cells in predominant fibromatous stromal component

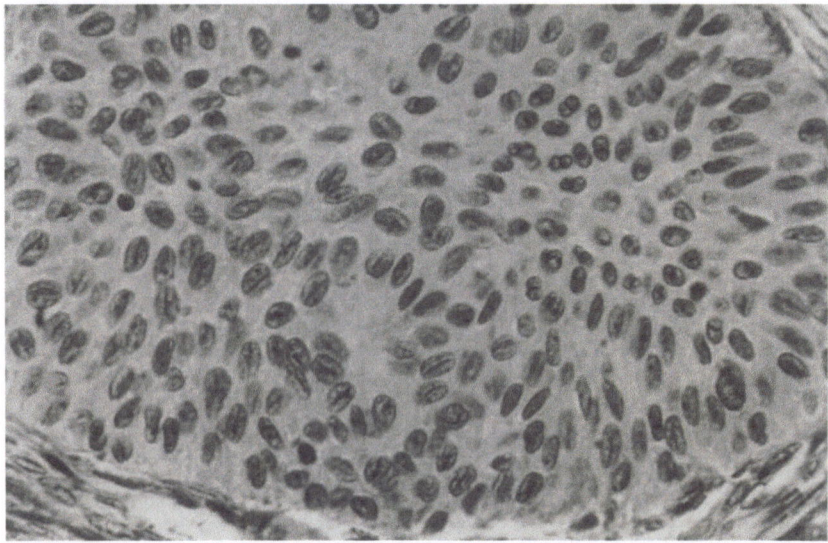

Fig. 48. *Brenner tumour.* Nests of transitional cells, many containing coffee-bean nuclei with longitudinal grooves. [From Scully RE, Young RH, Clement PB (1998) Tumors of the ovary, maldeveloped gonads, fallopian tube, and broad ligament. Atlas of tumor pathology, 3rd series. Armed Forces Institute of Pathology, Washington, DC]

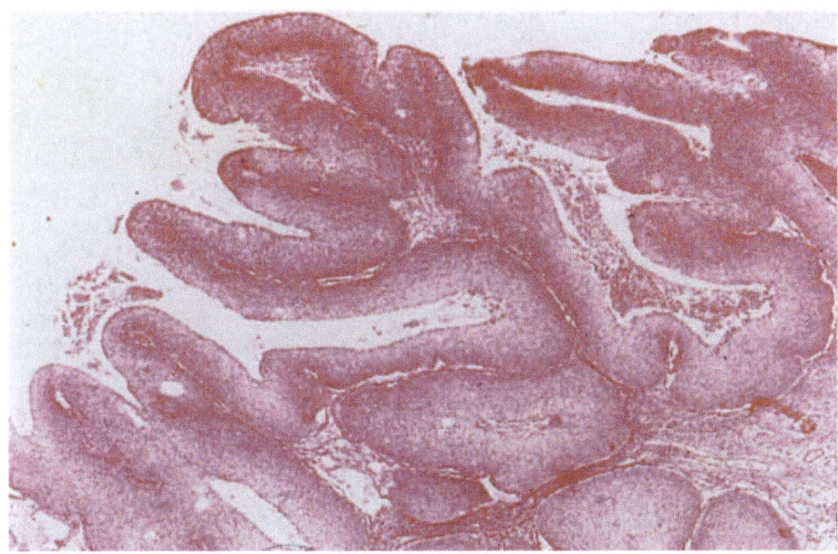

Fig. 49. *Brenner tumour of borderline malignancy.* Cysts lined by branching papillae covered by atypical transitional epithelium

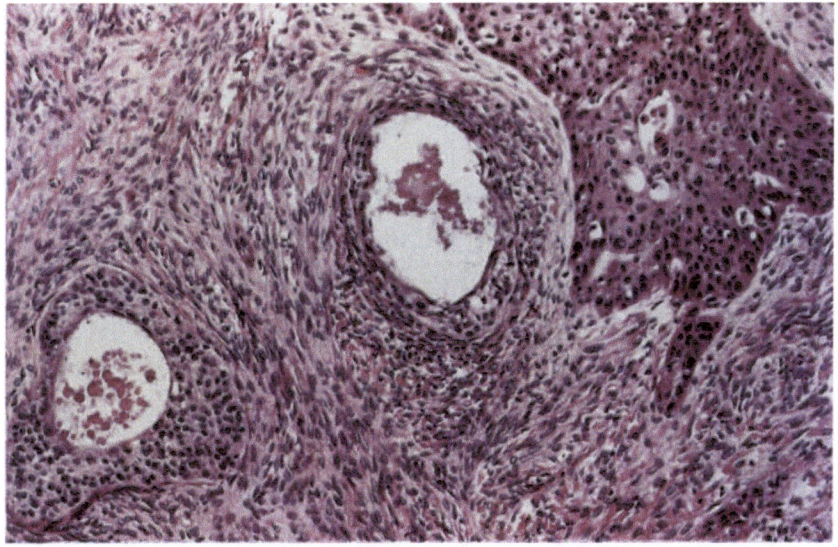

Fig. 50. *Malignant Brenner tumour.* Two cystic benign Brenner nests and single irregular carcinomatous aggregate lying in fibromatous stromal component

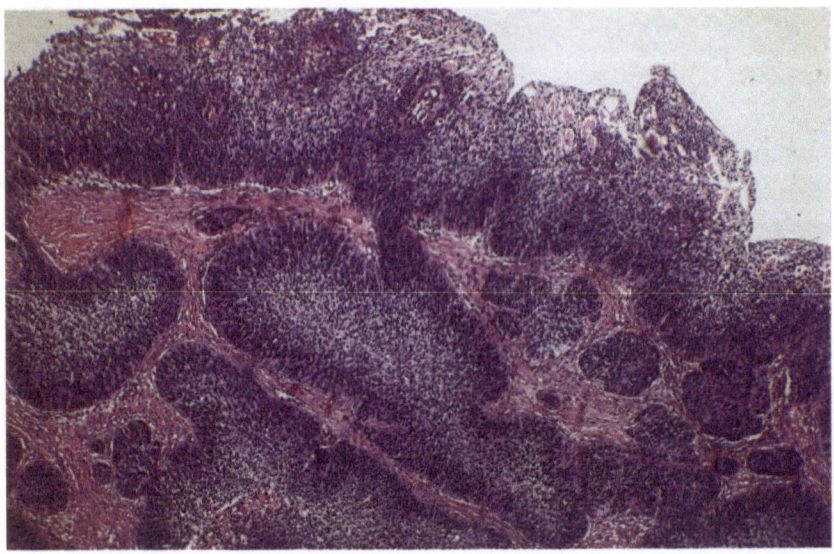

Fig. 51. *Transitional cell carcinoma.* Cyst lined by malignant transitional epithelium invading stroma in irregular rounded nests

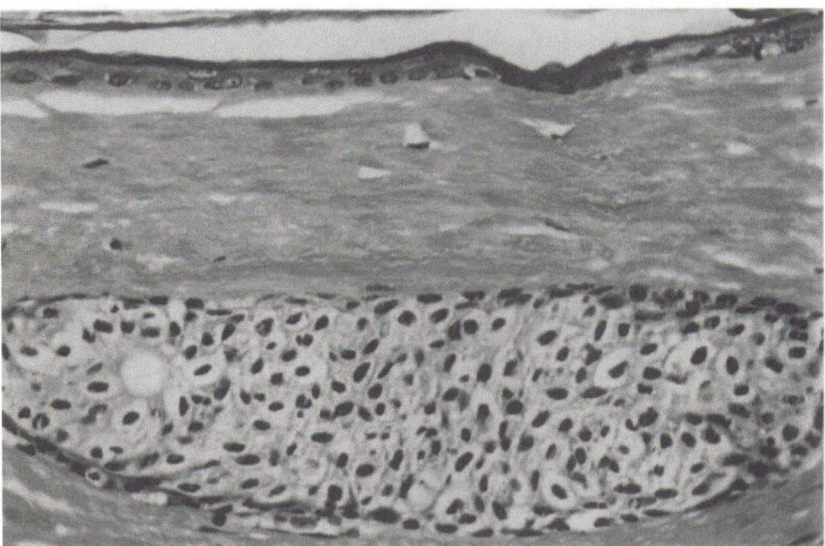

Fig. 52. *Epidermoid cyst.* Cyst lined by keratinizing squamous epithelium and nest resembling Walthard nests in wall of cyst. [From Young RH, Prat J, Scully RE (1980) Epidermoid cyst of the ovary. A report of three cases with comments on histogenesis. Am J Clin Pathol 73:273–276]

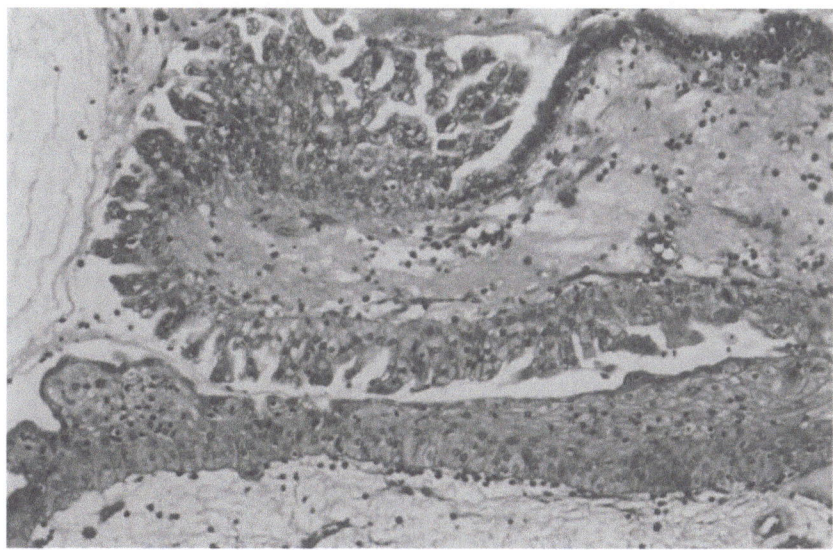

Fig. 53. *Papillary cystic tumour of borderline malignancy of mixed cell types.* Squamous epithelium and mucinous epithelium with cellular budding. [From Scully RE, Young RH, Clement PB (1998) Tumors of the ovary, maldeveloped gonads, fallopian tube, and broad ligament. Atlas of tumor pathology, 3rd series. Armed Forces Institute of Pathology, Washington, DC]

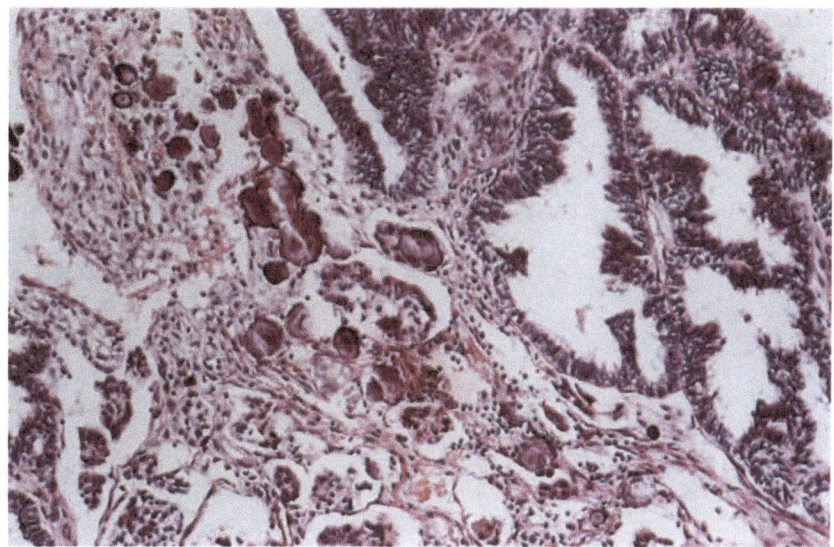

Fig. 54. *Serous papillary carcinoma (left) and endometrioid adenocarcinoma (right).* Papillary carcinoma with psammoma bodies and endometrioid glands. [From Scully RE, Young RH, Clement PB (1998) Tumors of the ovary, maldeveloped gonads, fallopian tube, and broad ligament. Atlas of tumor pathology, 3rd series. Armed Forces Institute of Pathology, Washington, DC]

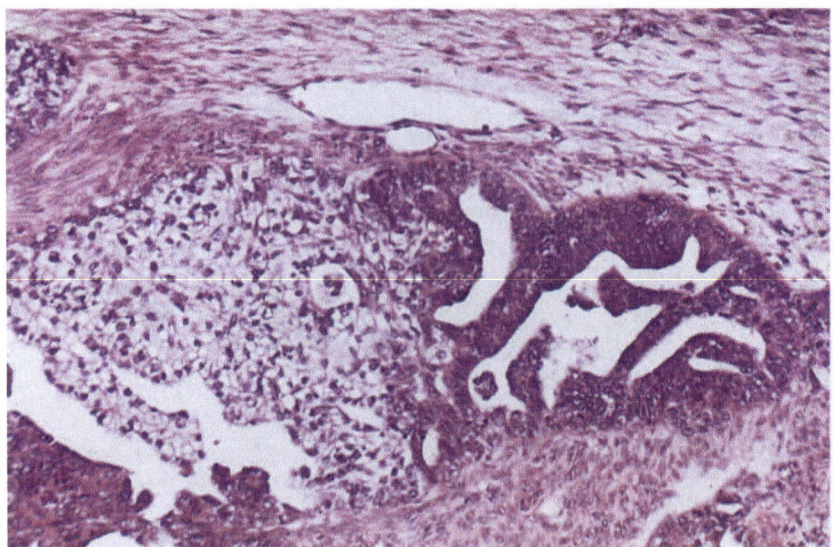

Fig. 55. *Clear cell carcinoma (left) and endometrioid adenocarcinoma (right), mixed.* Solid area of clear cell carcinoma juxtaposed to malignant endometrioid glands

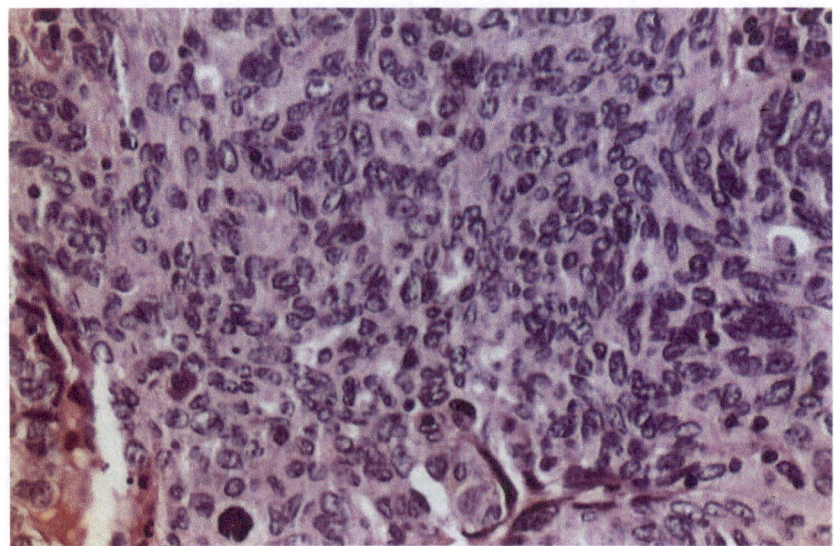

Fig. 56. *Undifferentiated carcinoma.* Poorly differentiated cells with scanty cytoplasm and highly atypical nuclei

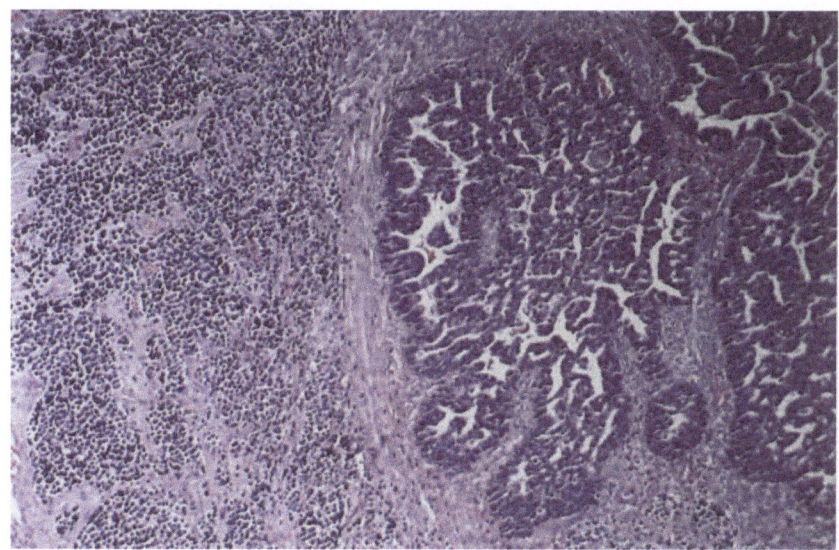

Fig. 57. *Undifferentiated carcinoma, pulmonary small cell type.* Component of endometrioid adenocarcinoma adjacent to small cell carcinoma

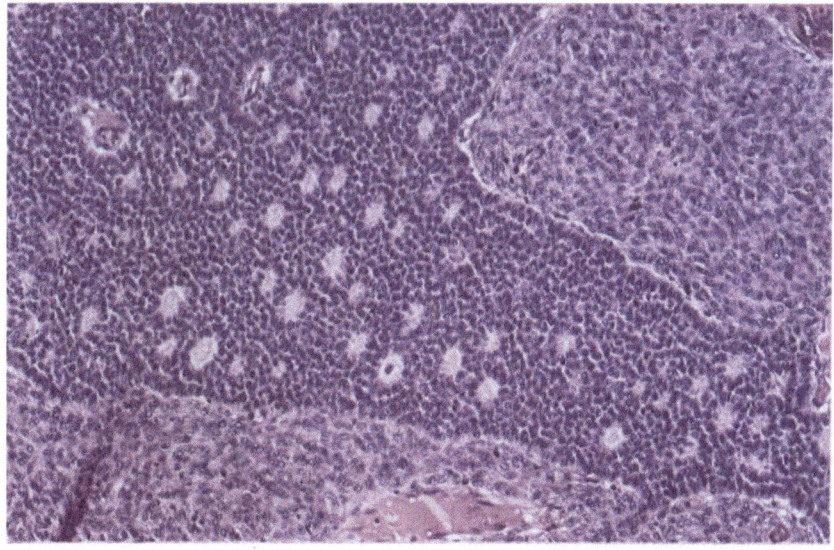

Fig. 58. *Granulosa cell tumour, adult type.* Microfollicular pattern with Call-Exner bodies. [From Scully RE, Young RH, Clement PB (1998) Tumors of the ovary, mal-developed gonads, fallopian tube, and broad ligament. Atlas of tumor pathology, 3rd series. Armed Forces Institute of Pathology, Washington, DC]

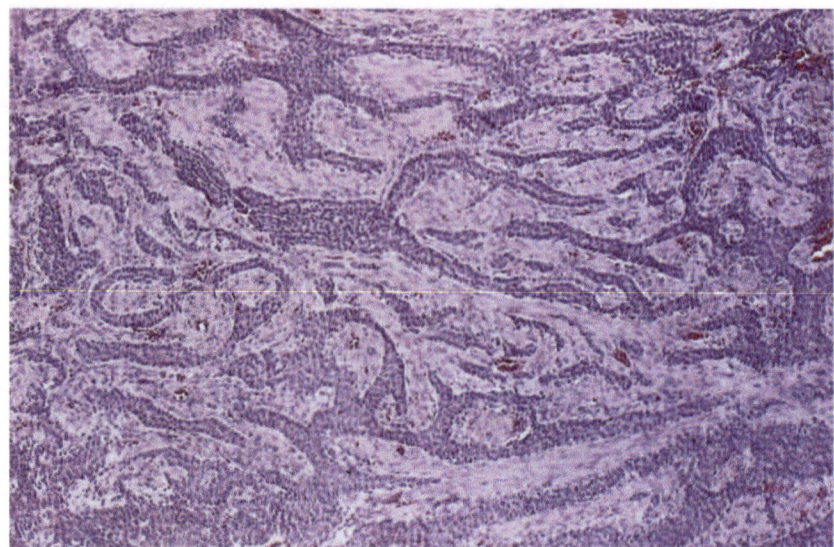

Fig. 59. *Granulosa cell tumour, adult type.* Trabecular pattern with trabeculae separated by fibrothecomatous component

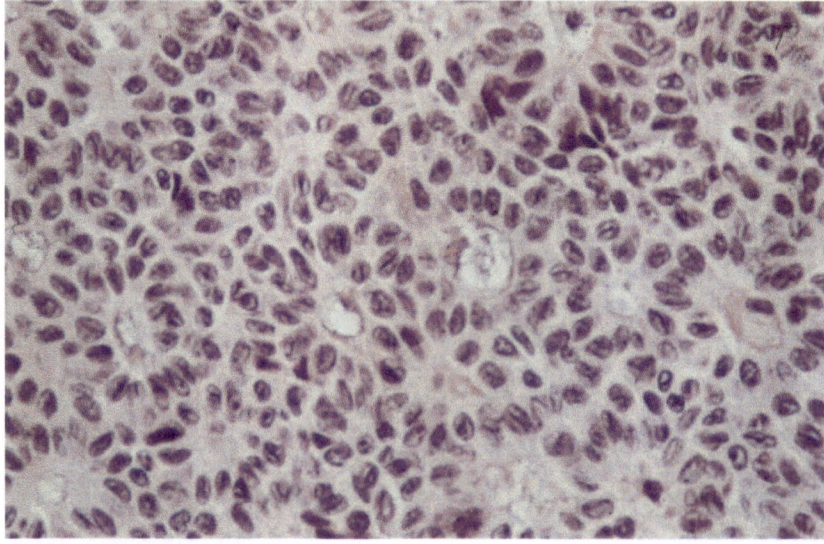

Fig. 60. *Granulosa cell tumour, adult type.* Pale angular nuclei, some of which have grooves

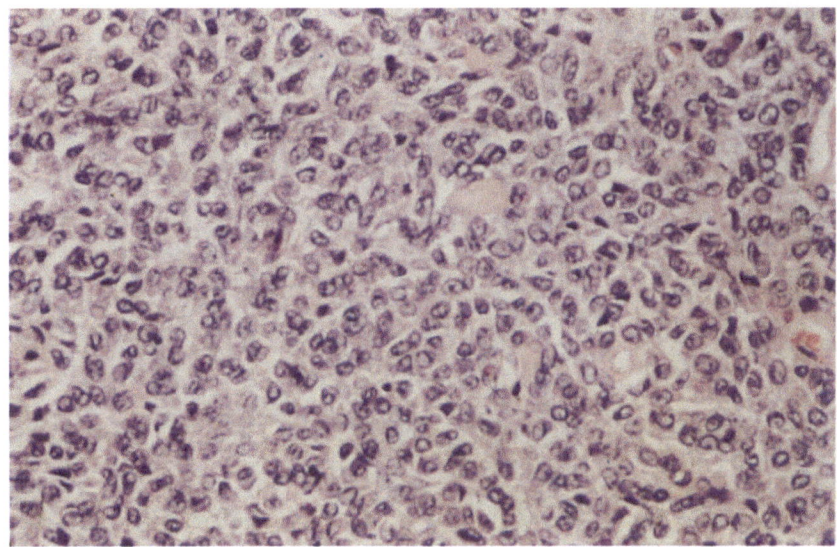

Fig. 61. *Granulosa cell tumour, adult type.* Diffuse arrangement of cells with uniform pale, rounded nuclei

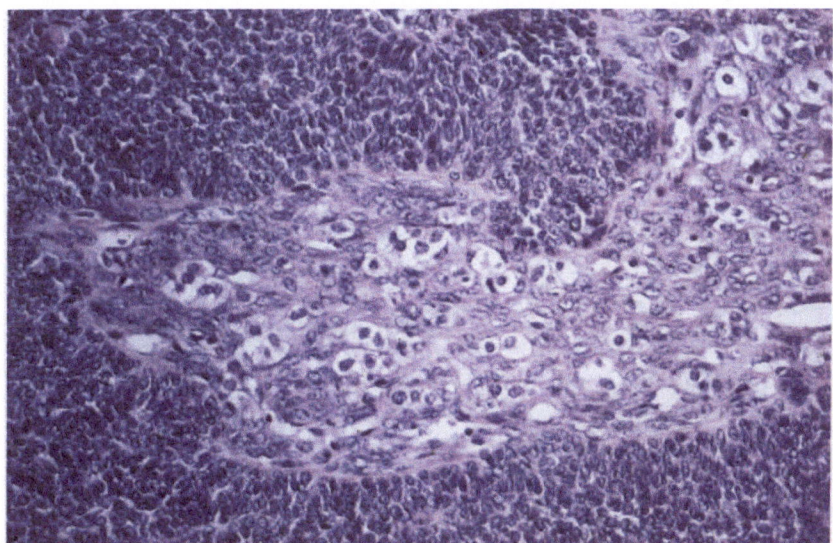

Fig. 62. *Granulosa cell tumour, adult type.* Trabeculae of granulosa cells separated by fibrothecomatous stromal component containing lipid rich, pale theca cells

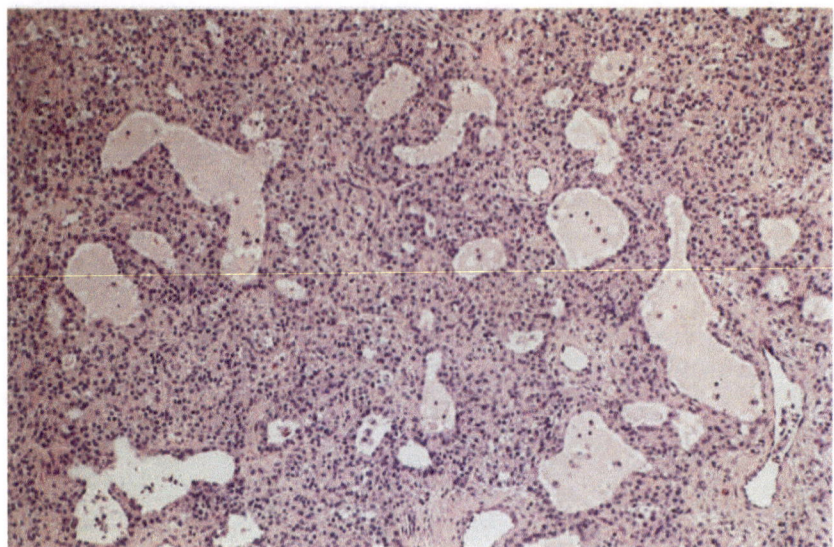

Fig. 63. *Granulosa cell tumour, juvenile type.* Diffuse arrangement of tumour cells punctured by follicles of variable size and shape

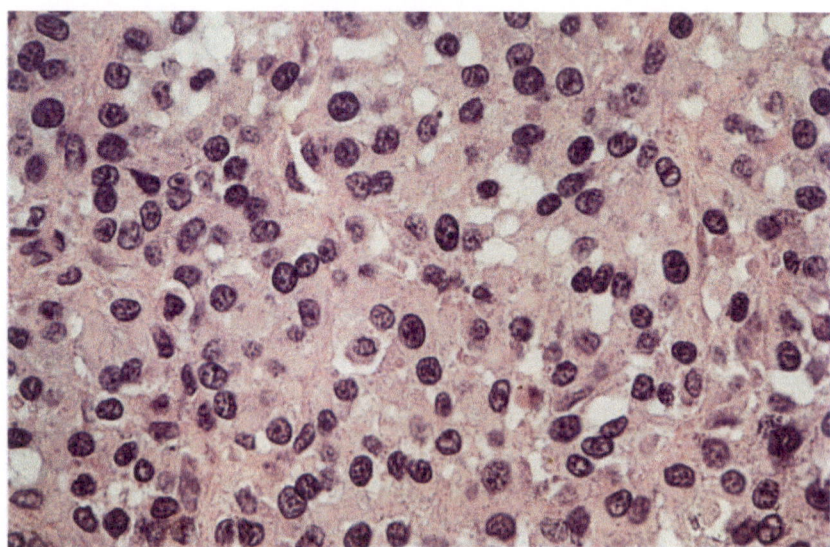

Fig. 64. *Granulosa cell tumour, juvenile type.* Cells containing abundant eosinophilic cytoplasm (luteinized cells) with round, moderately dark nuclei

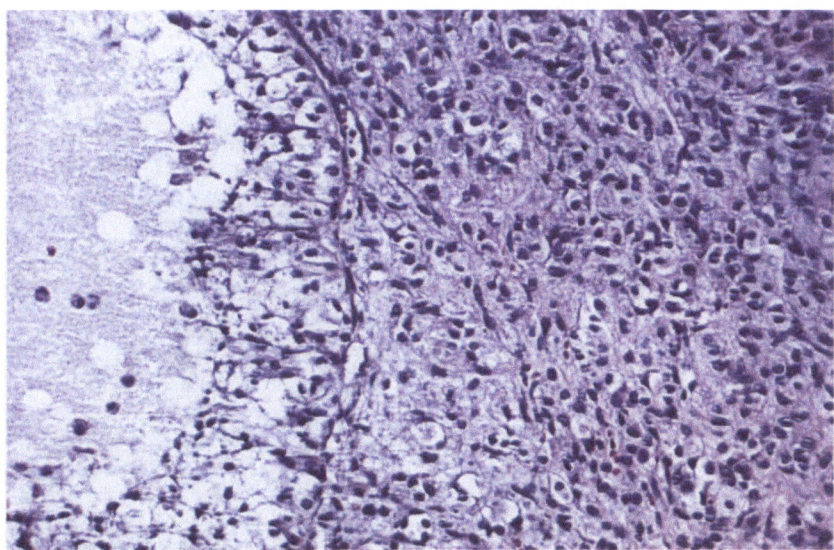

Fig. 65. *Granulosa cell tumour, juvenile type.* Luteinized, lipid-containing theca cells and granulosa cells lining follicle. [From Scully RE, Young RH, Clement PB (1998) Tumors of the ovary, maldeveloped gonads, fallopian tube, and broad ligament. Atlas of tumor pathology, 3rd series. Armed Forces Institute of Pathology, Washington, DC]

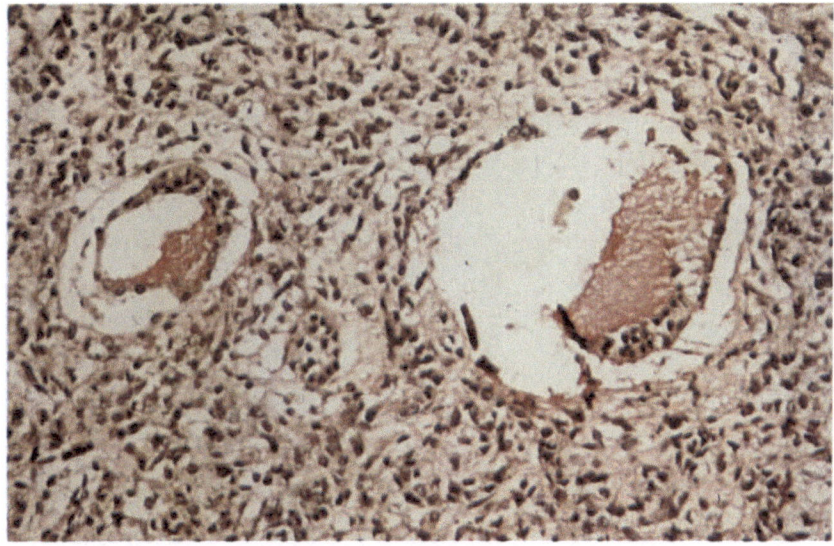

Fig. 66. *Granulosa cell tumour, juvenile type.* Mucinous follicular fluid. Mucicarmine stain. [From Scully RE, Young RH, Clement PB (1998) Tumors of the ovary, maldeveloped gonads, fallopian tube, and broad ligament. Atlas of tumor pathology, 3rd series. Armed Forces Institute of Pathology, Washington, DC]

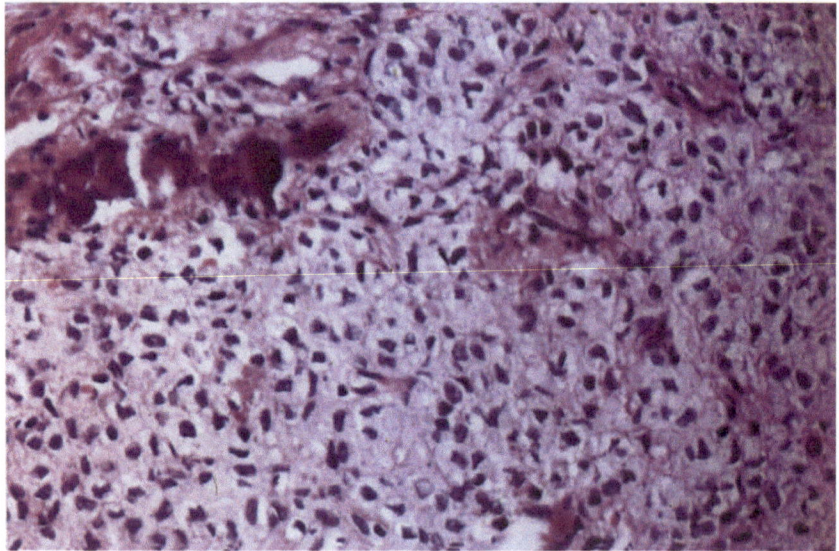

Fig. 67. *Thecoma.* Cells containing abundant lipid-rich cytoplasm with focal calcification

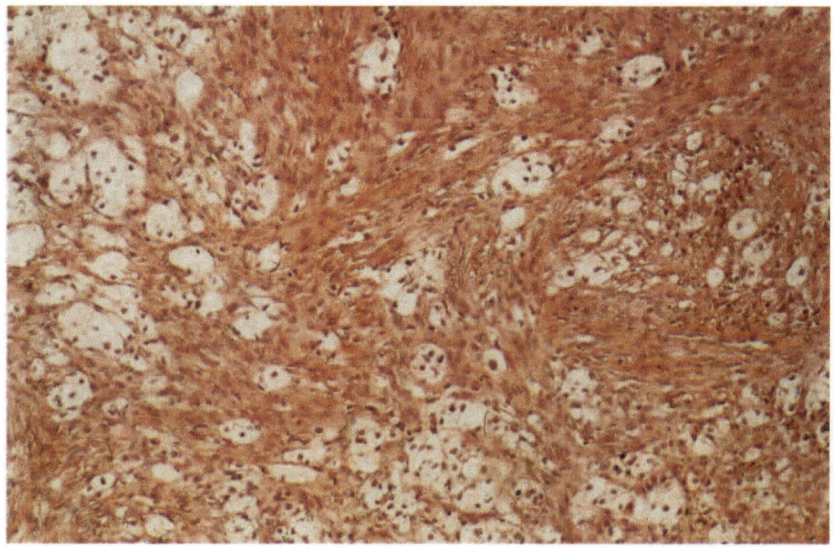

Fig. 68. *Luteinized thecoma.* Islands of lipid-rich lutein cells on a fibromatous background

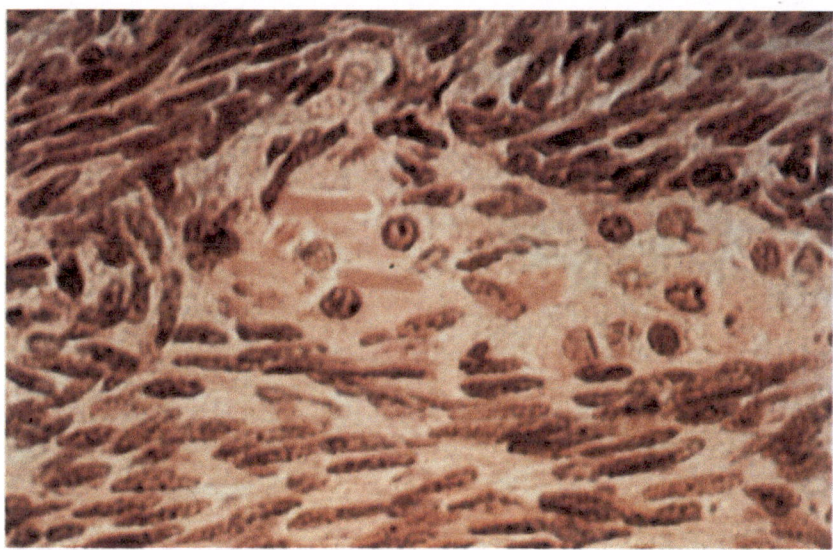

Fig. 69. *Stromal Leydig cell tumour.* Nest of Leydig cells containing crystals of Reinke on a fibromatous background. [From Scully RE, Young RH, Clement PB (1998) Tumors of the ovary, maldeveloped gonads, fallopian tube, and broad ligament. Atlas of tumor pathology, 3rd series. Armed Forces Institute of Pathology, Washington, DC]

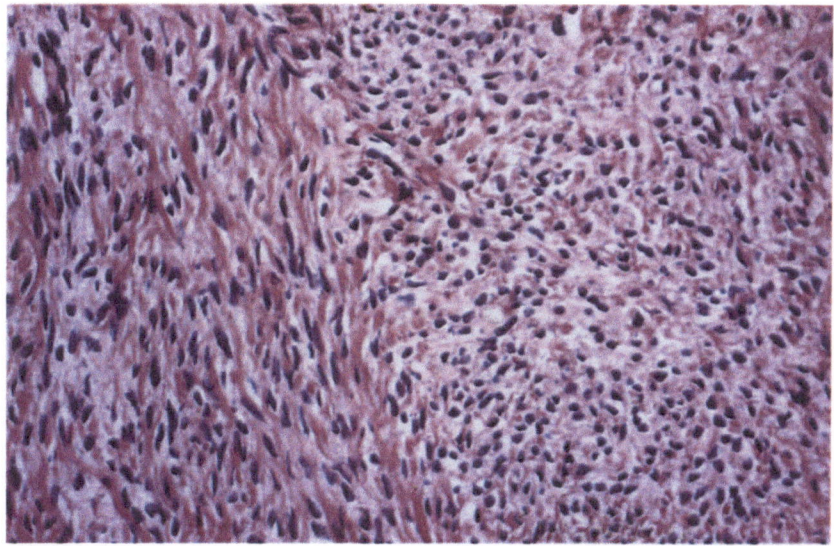

Fig. 70. *Fibroma.* Intersecting fascicles of spindle cells that have produced collagen

90

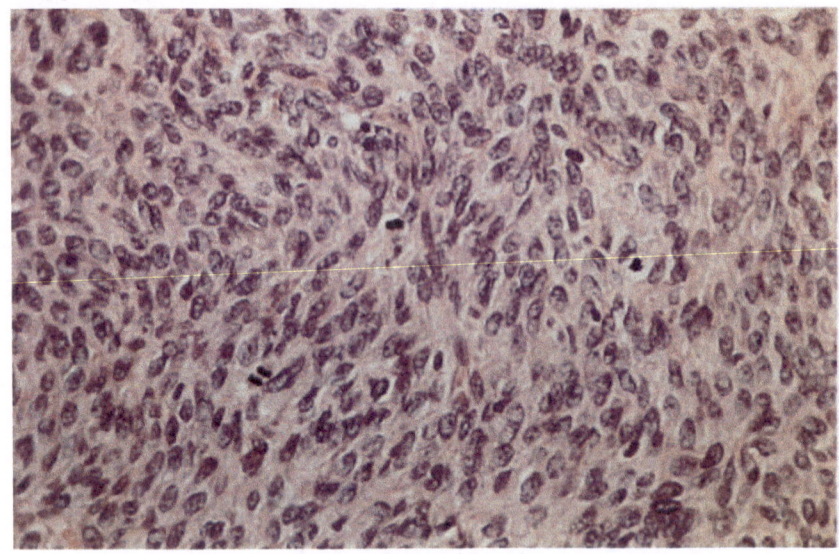

Fig. 71. *Cellular fibroma.* Crowded spindle cells without atypical nuclei with one mitotic figure

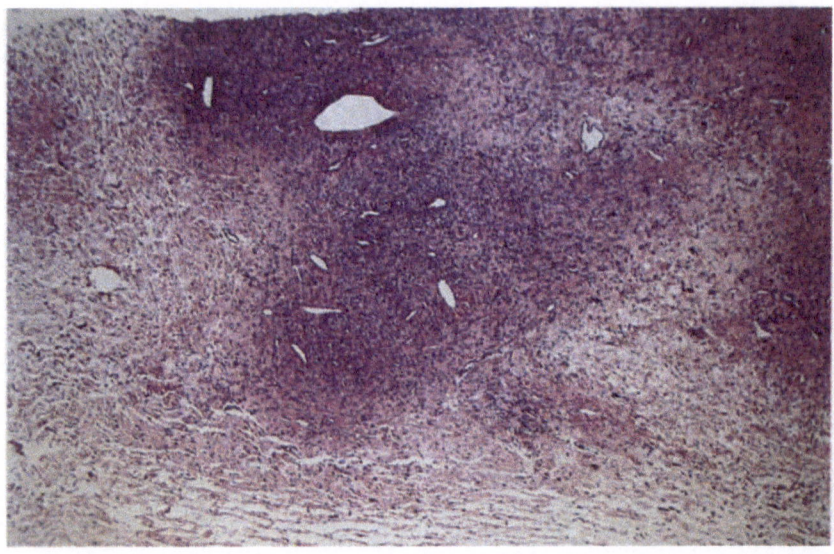

Fig. 72. *Sclerosing stromcl tumour.* Cellular, well-vascularized pseudolobule surrounded by oedematous collagenous component

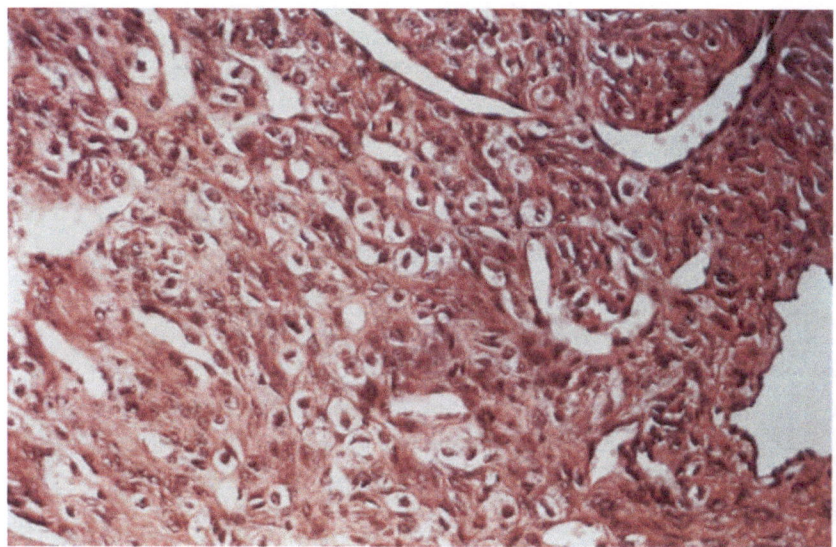

Fig. 73. *Sclerosing stromal tumour.* Disorderly arrangement of large clear cells with shrunken nuclei and spindle cells that have produced collagen; abundant vessels

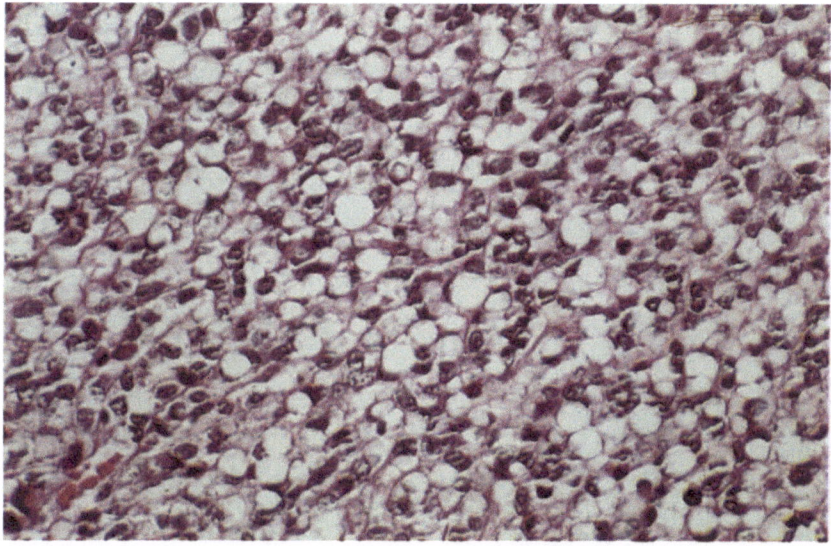

Fig. 74. *Signet-ring stromal tumour.* Cytoplasm distended by empty vacuoles with eccentric displacement of nuclei

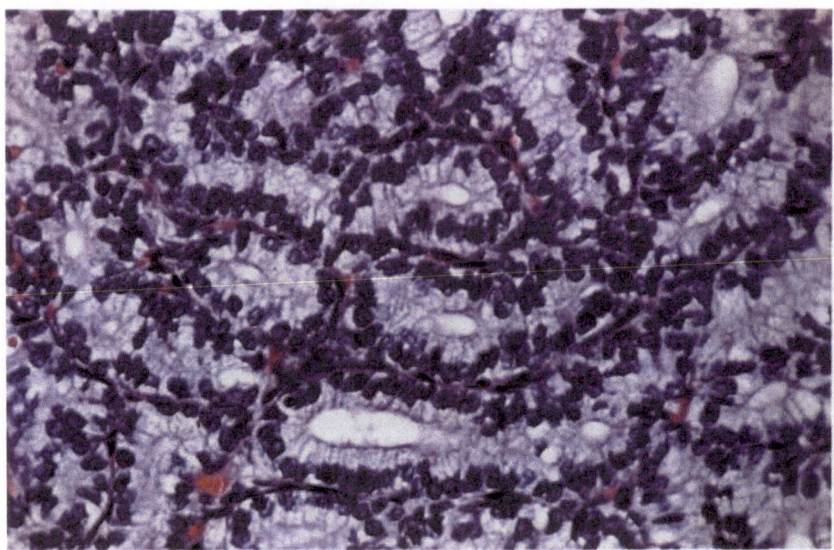

Fig. 75. *Sertoli cell tumour.* Crowded tubules with lumens lined by vacuolated, lipid-rich cytoplasm

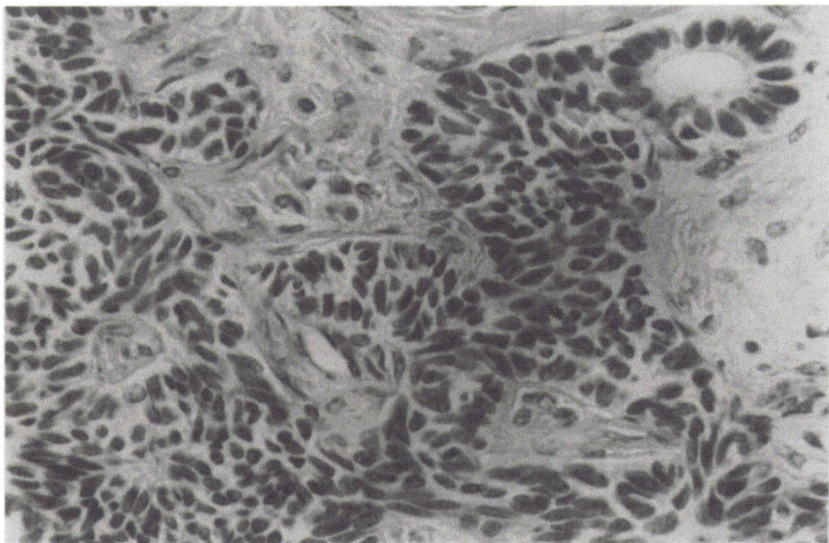

Fig. 76. *Sertoli cell tumour.* Hollow tubule merging with anastomosing trabeculae composed of spindle-shaped Sertoli cells

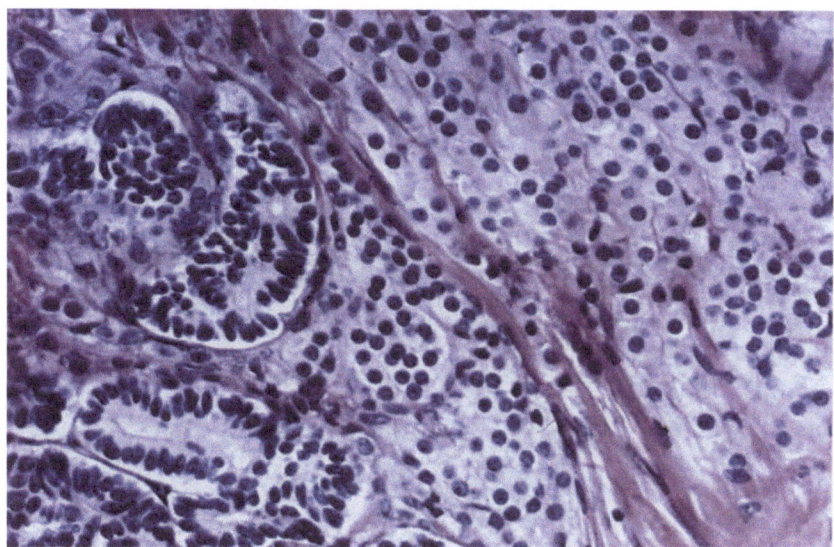

Fig. 77. *Sertoli-Leydig cell tumour, well differentiated.* Leydig cells (*right*) and hollow tubules (*left*)

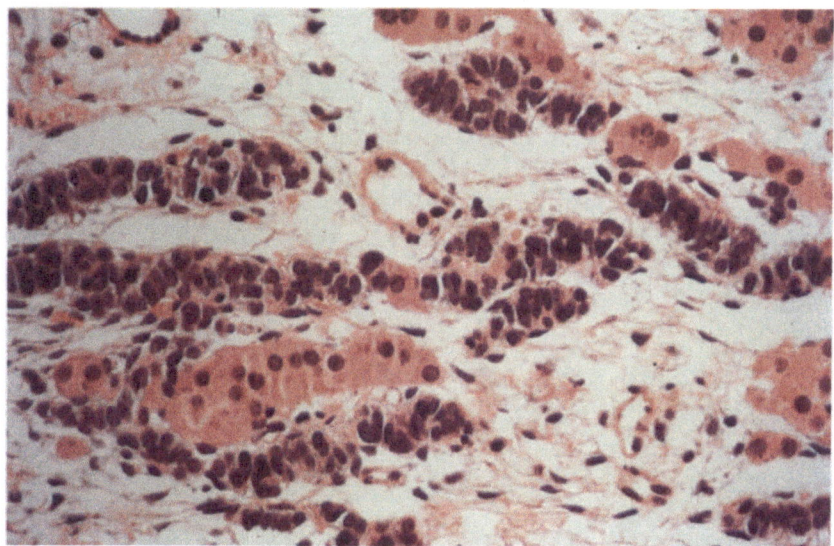

Fig. 78. *Sertoli-Leydig cell tumour, intermediate.* Sex cords composed of immature Sertoli cells and aggregates of Leydig cells with abundant eosinophilic cytoplasm. [From Young, RH, Clement PB, Scully RE (1994) The ovary. In: Sternberg SS (ed) Diagnostic surgical pathology. Raven, New York, pp 2195–2279]

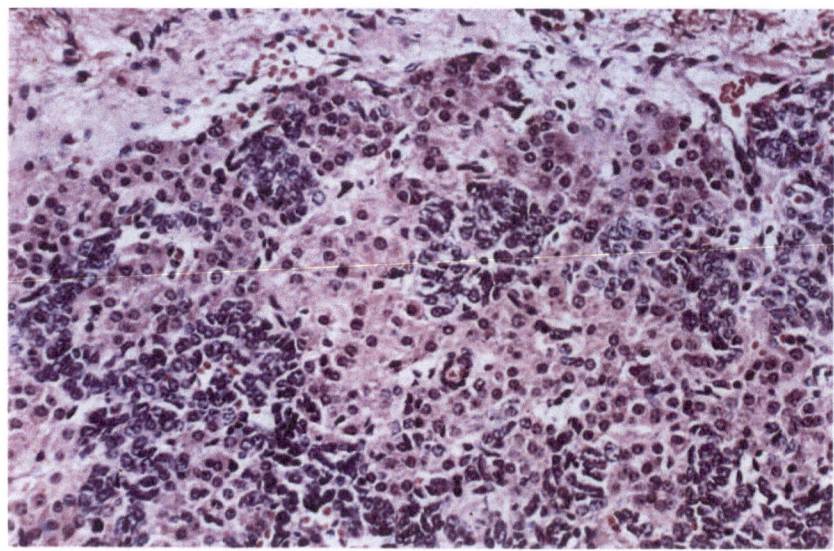

Fig. 79. *Sertoli-Leydig cell tumour, intermediate.* Interconnected groups of Sertoli cells with dark nuclei separated by Leydig cells with abundant eosinophilic cytoplasm

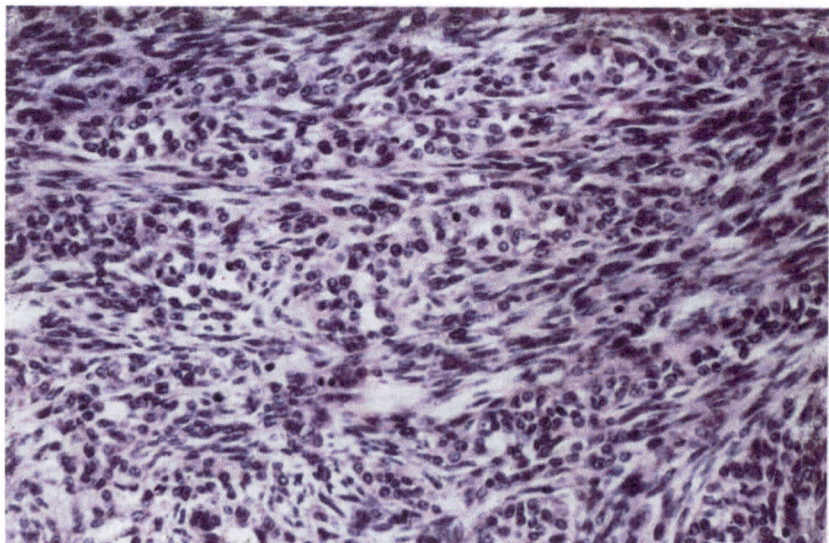

Fig. 80. *Sertoli-Leydig cell tumour, poorly differentiated.* Fibrosarcomatoid pattern with scattered rounded cells with abundant cytoplasm resembling Leydig cells

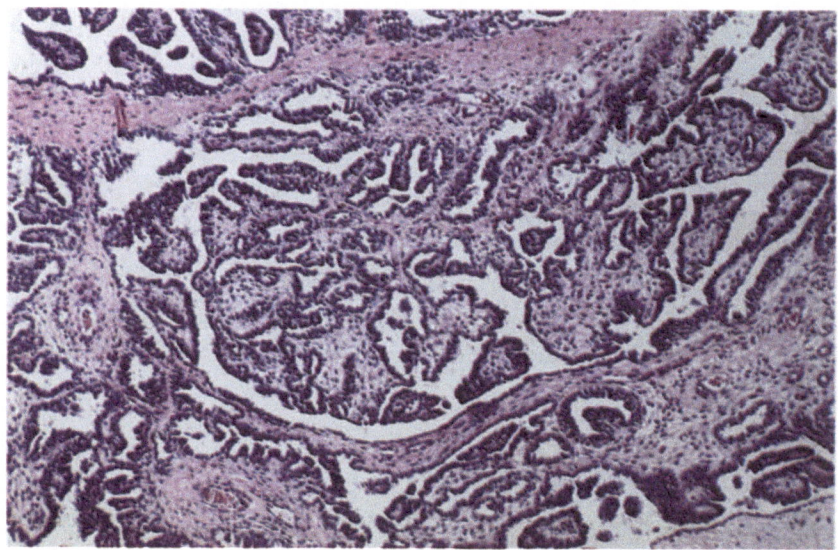

Fig. 81. *Retiform Sertoli-Leydig cell tumour.* Network of tubules with papillae lined by stratified epithelium

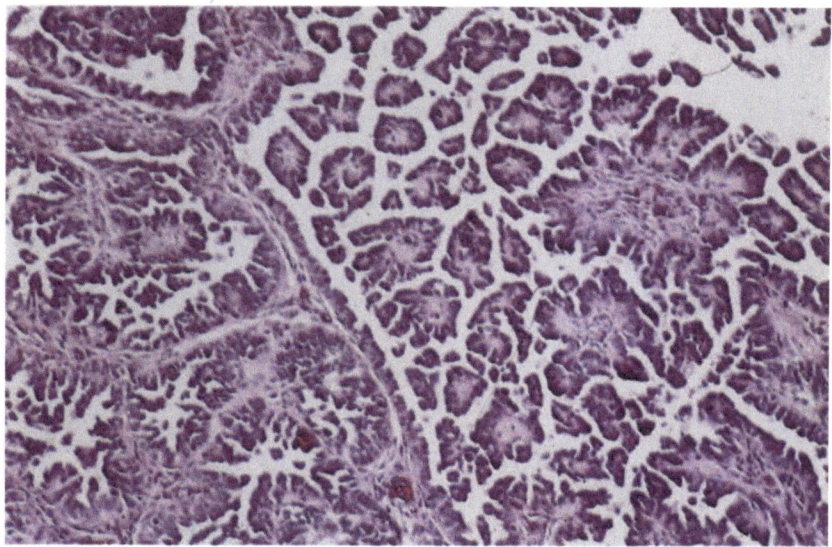

Fig. 82. *Retiform Sertoli-Leydig cell tumour.* Papillary pattern resembling that of serous borderline tumour

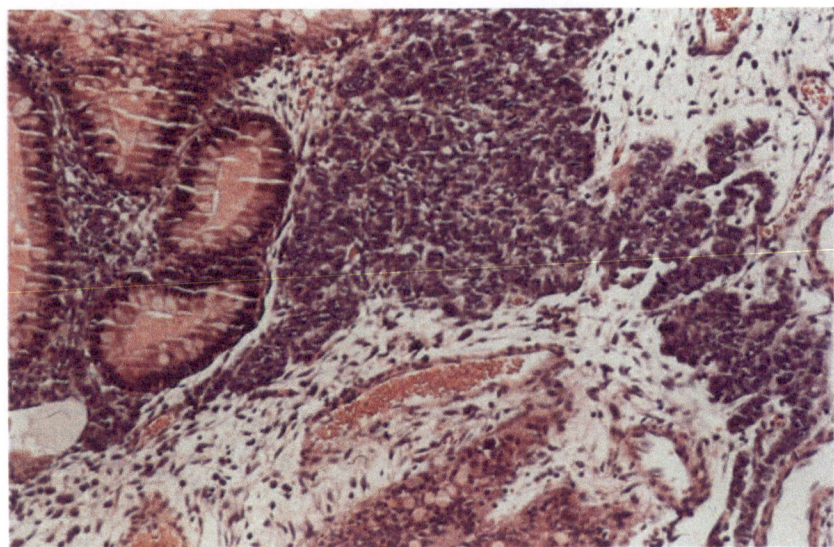

Fig. 83. *Sertoli-Leydig cell tumour, intermediate, with heterologous elements.* Glands lined by intestinal-type epithelium adjacent to nests and cords of immature Sertoli cells

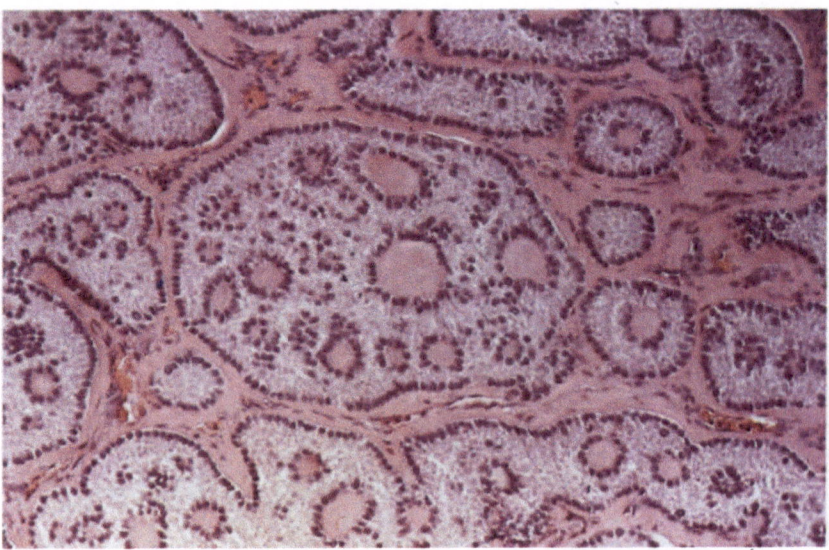

Fig. 84. *Sex cord tumour with annular tubules.* Simple and complex annular tubules surrounding rounded hyaline nodules. [From Scully RE, Young RH, Clement PB (1998) Tumors of the ovary, maldeveloped gonads, fallopian tube, and broad ligament. Atlas of tumor pathology, 3rd series. Armed Forces Institute of Pathology, Washington, DC]

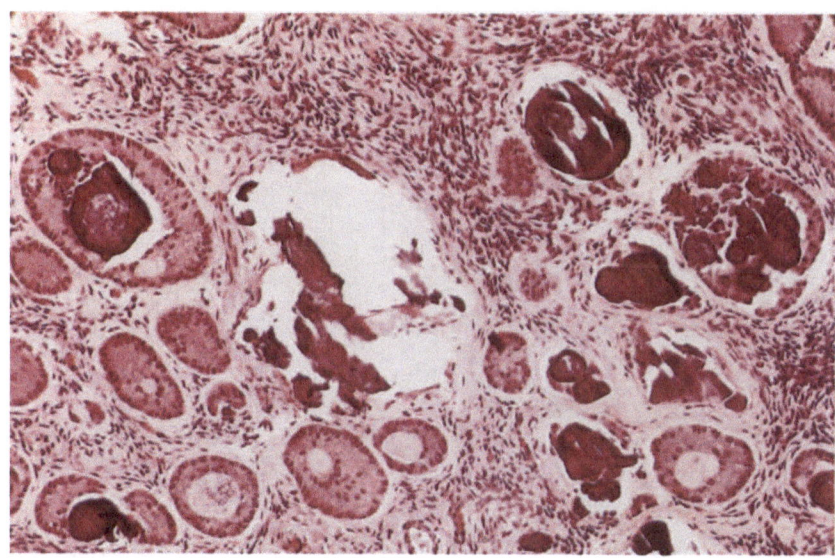

Fig. 85. *Sex cord tumour with annular tubules.* Extensive calcification in tumour from patient with Peutz-Jeghers syndrome

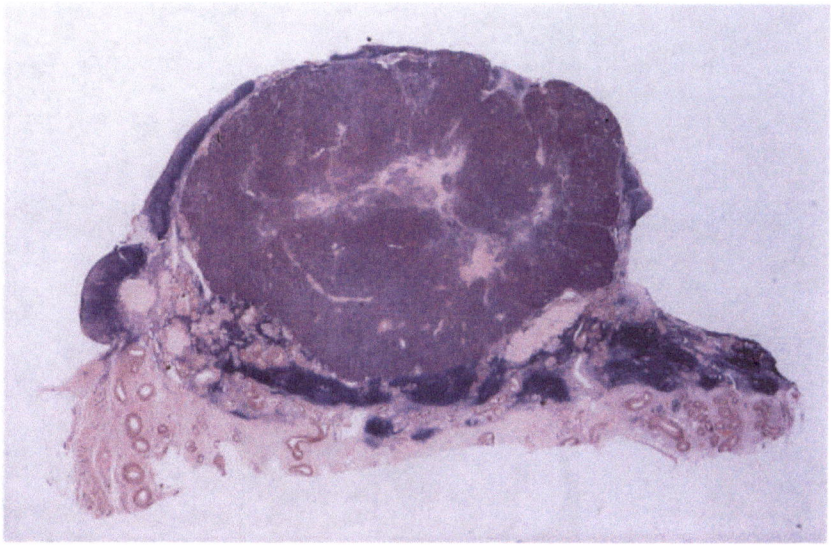

Fig. 86. *Stromal luteoma.* Steroid cell tumour surrounded by thin rim of ovarian stroma. [From Scully RE, Young RH, Clement PB (1998) Tumors of the ovary, maldeveloped gonads, fallopian tube, and broad ligament. Atlas of tumor pathology, 3rd series. Armed Forces Institute of Pathology, Washington, DC]

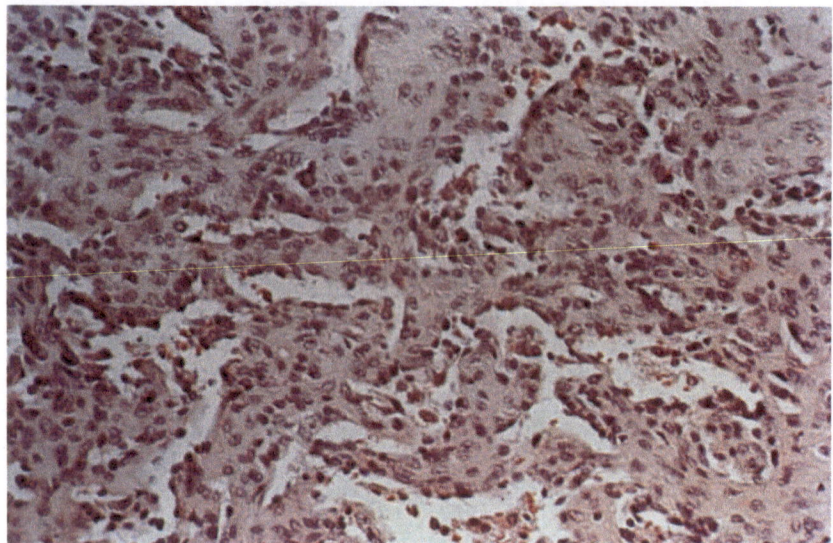

Fig. 87. *Stromal luteoma.* Degenerative changes simulating pattern of vascular tumour

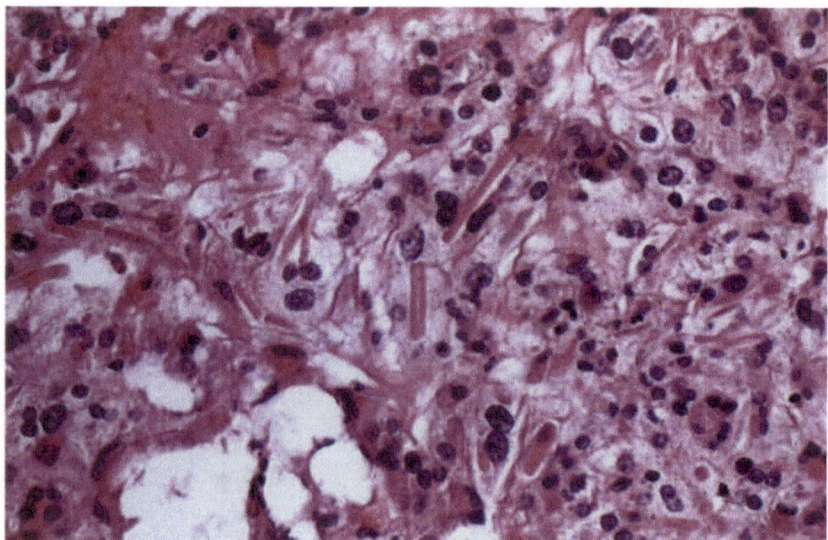

Fig. 88. *Leydig cell tumour.* Cells containing crystals of Reinke. [From Young RH, Clement PB, Scully RE (1994) The ovary. In: Sternberg SS (ed) Diagnostic surgical pathology. Raven, New York, pp 2195–2279

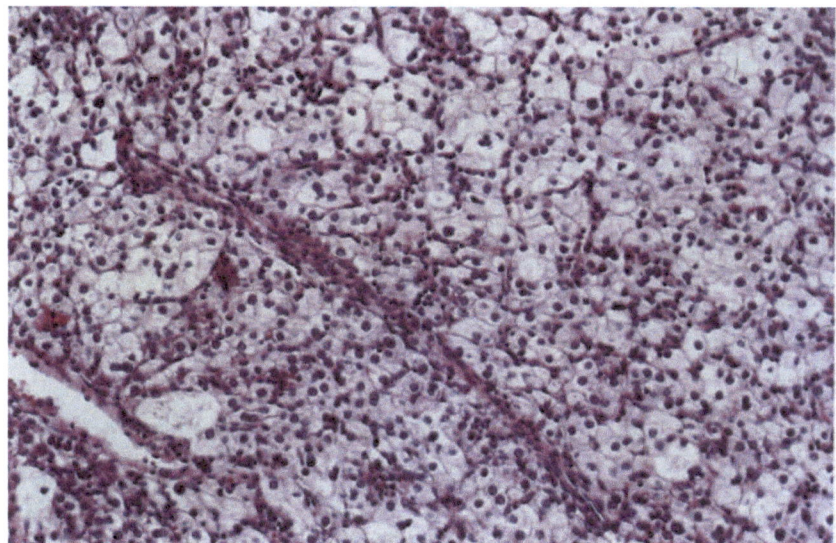

Fig. 89. *Steroid cell tumour, unclassified.* Lipid-rich cells

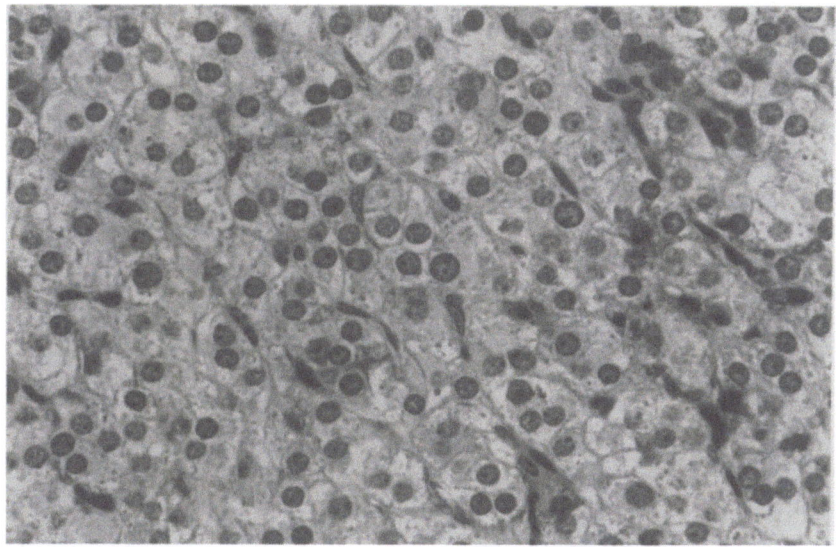

Fig. 90. *Steroid cell tumour, unclassified.* Lipid-poor cells with central nuclei and prominent nucleoli. [From Scully RE, Young RH, Clement PB (1998) Tumors of the ovary, maldeveloped gonads, fallopian tube, and broad ligament. Atlas of tumor pathology, 3rd series. Armed Forces Institute of Pathology, Washington, DC]

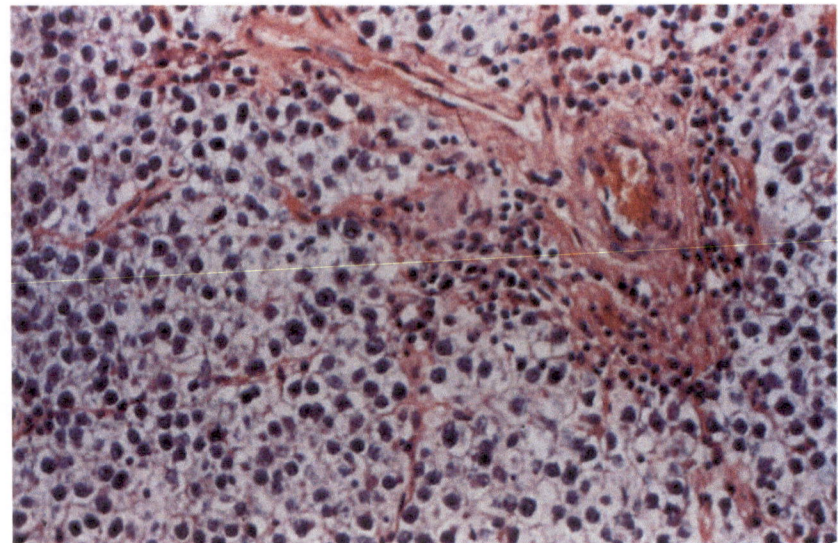

Fig. 91. *Dysgerminoma.* Diffuse arrangement of clear cells containing central rounded nuclei with lymphocytic infiltration of stroma

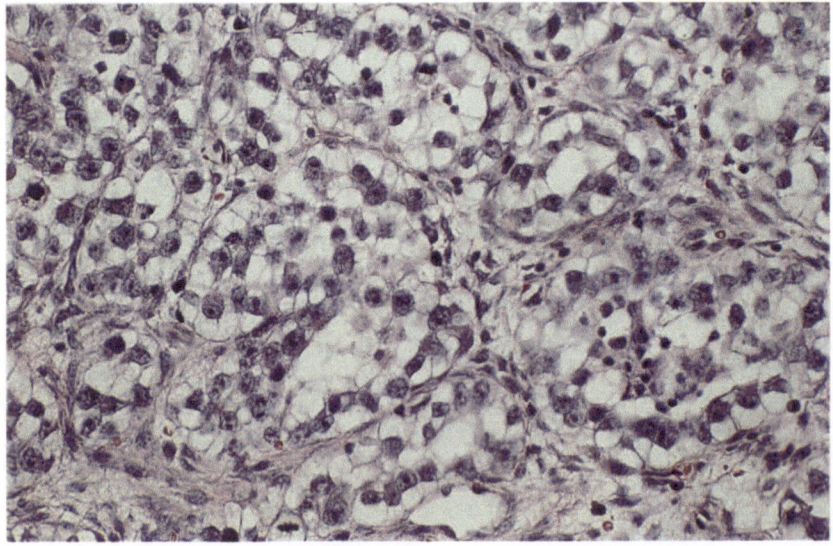

Fig. 92. *Dysgerminoma.* Flattened round nuclei with prominent nucleoli

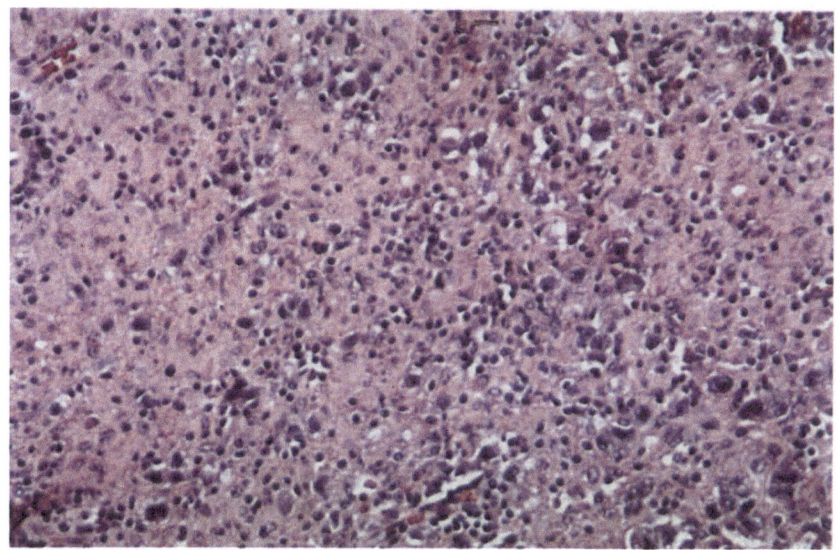

Fig. 93. *Dysgerminoma.* Extensive granulomatous reaction in stroma

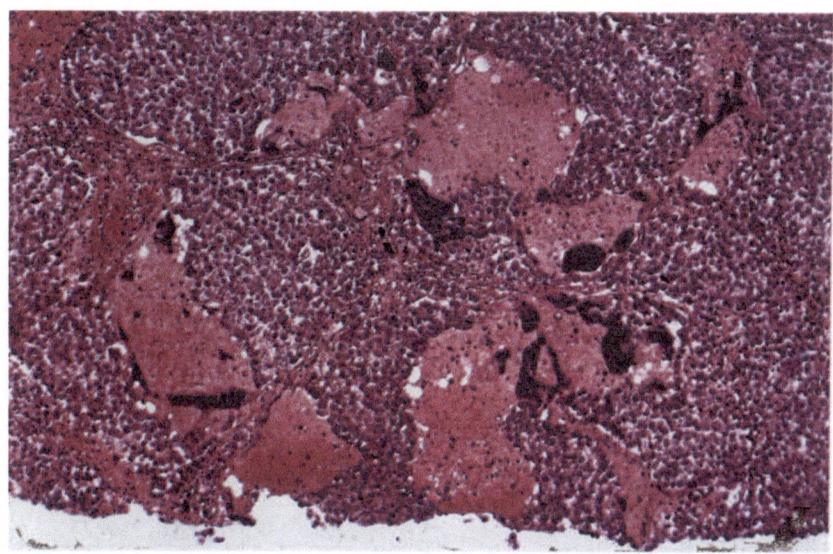

Fig. 94. *Dysgerminoma with syncytiotrophoblast cells.* Multinucleated cells adjacent to lakes of blood on background of dysgerminoma

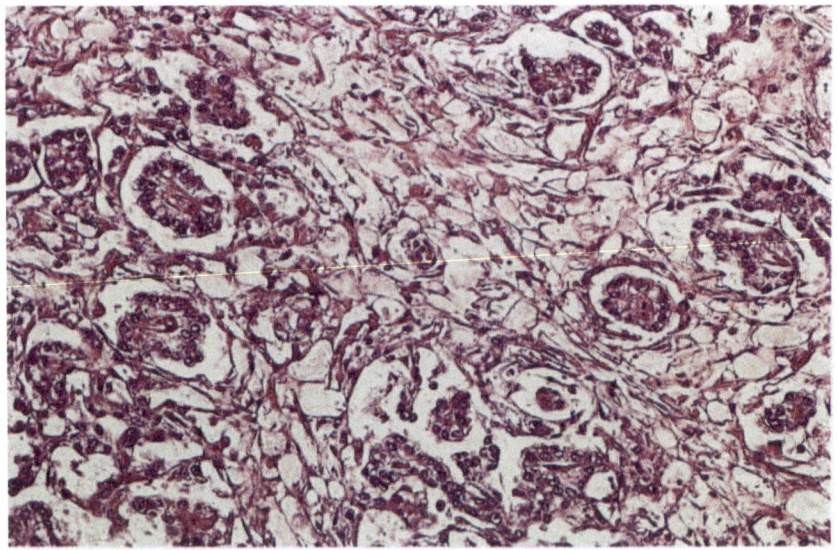

Fig. 95. *Yolk sac tumour.* Endodermal sinus pattern with Schiller-Duval bodies

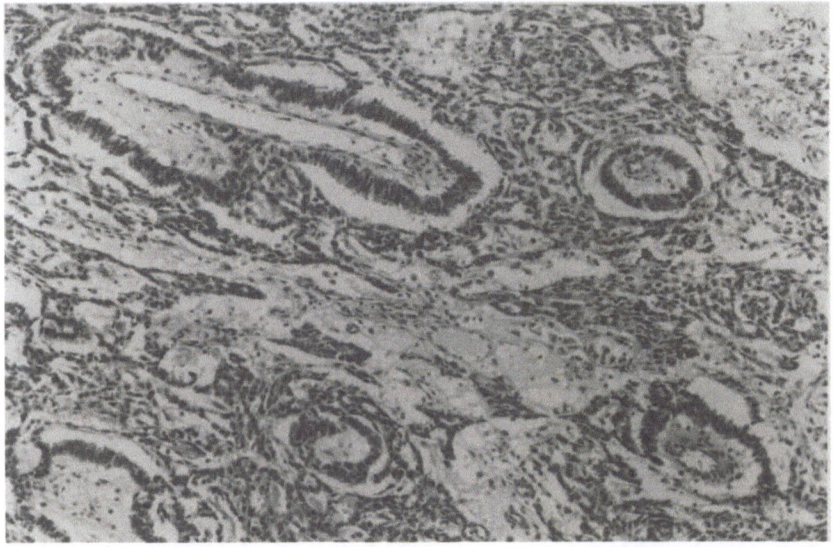

Fig. 96. *Yolk sac tumour.* Endodermal sinus pattern with Schiller-Duval bodies, one of which is elongated

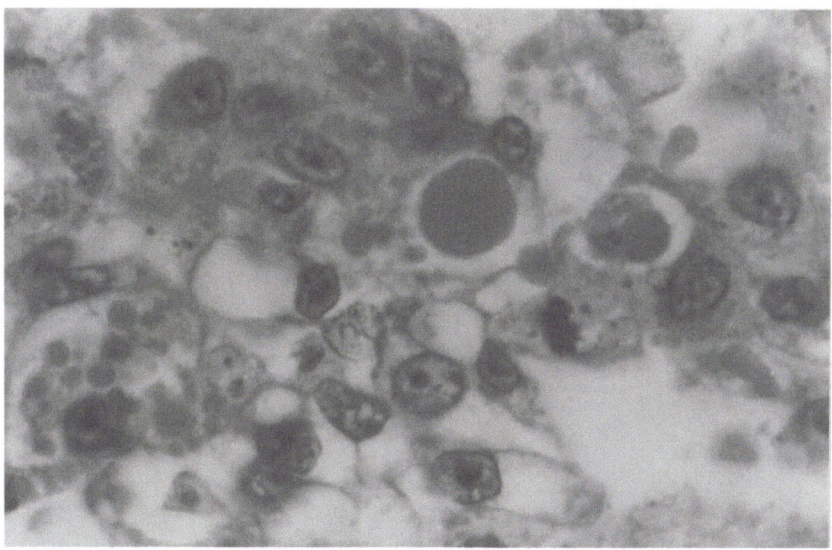

Fig. 97. *Yolk sac tumour.* Atypical nuclei, atypical mitotic figure and intracellular hyaline bodies

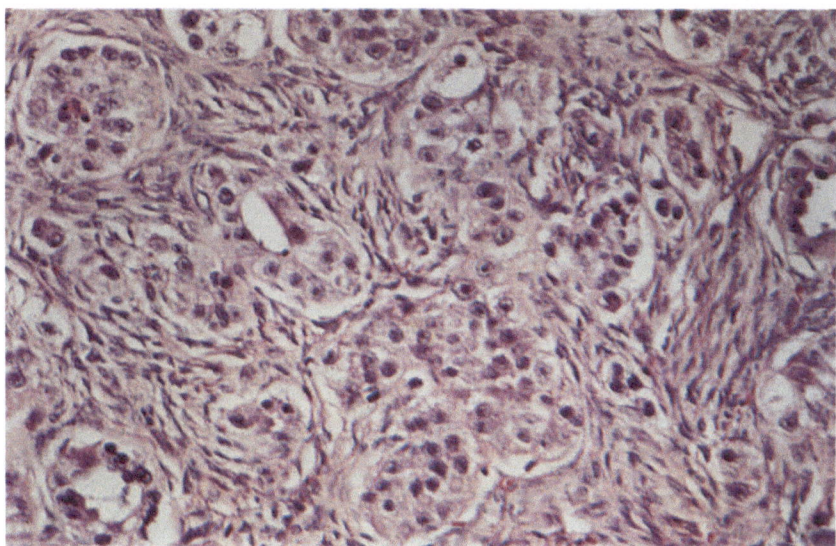

Fig. 98. *Yolk sac tumour.* Resemblance to dysgerminoma except for glandular spaces and absence of lymphocytes

104

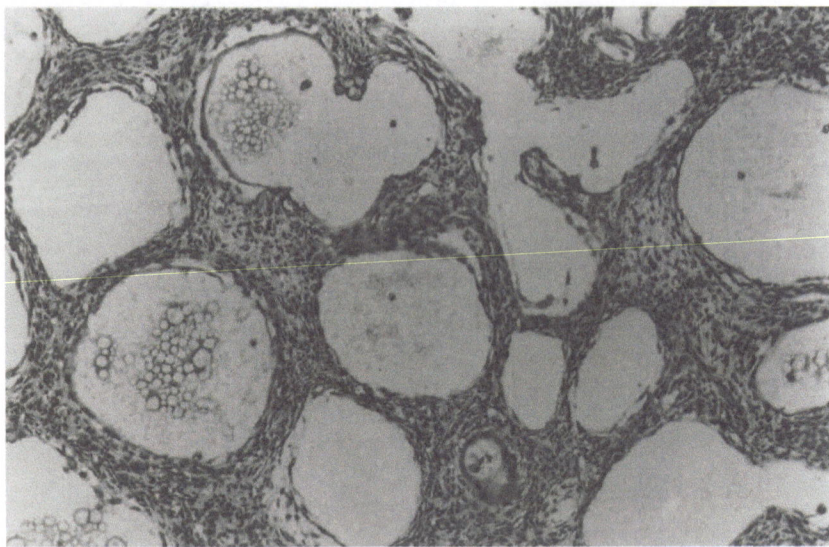

Fig. 99. *Yolk sac tumour, polyvesicular vitelline pattern.* Vesicles lined by flattened epithelium and separated by cellular mesenchyme

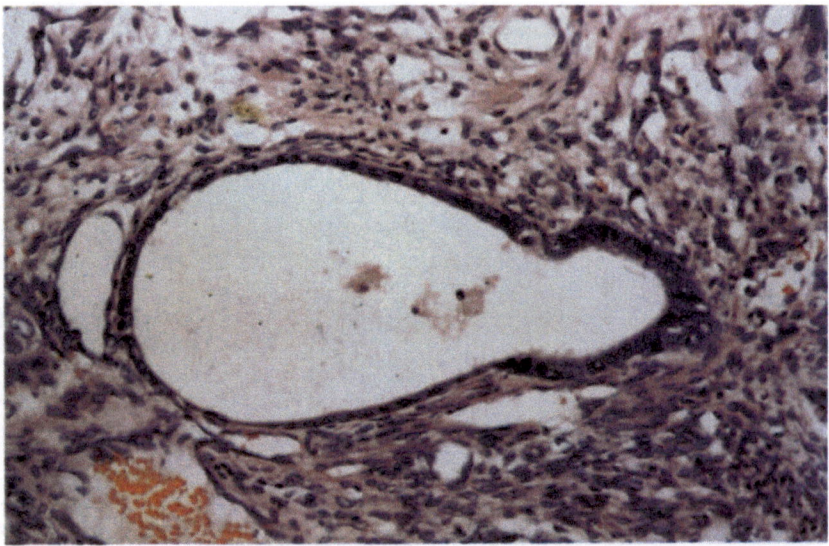

Fig. 100. *Yolk sac tumour, polyvesicular vitelline pattern.* Vesicle simulating normal embryonic division into primary vesicle lined by flat epithelium and secondary vesicle lined by columnar epithelium

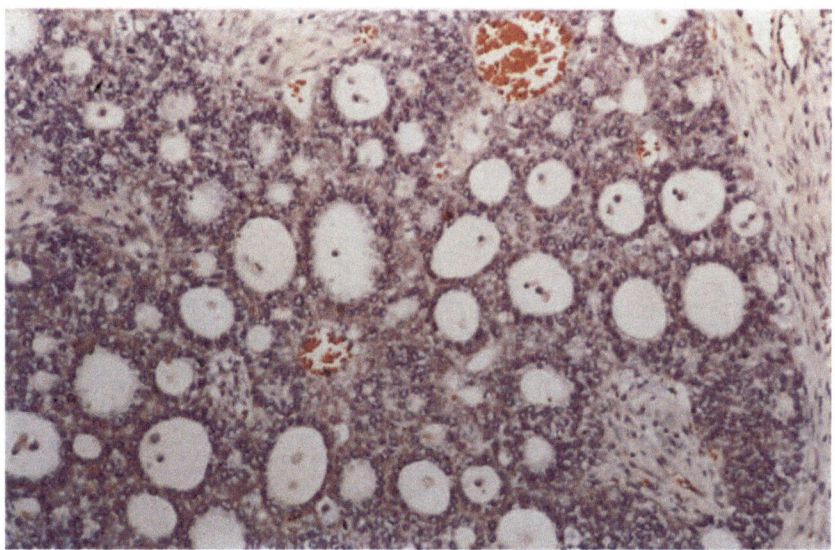

Fig. 101. *Glandular yolk sac tumour.* Cribriform pattern

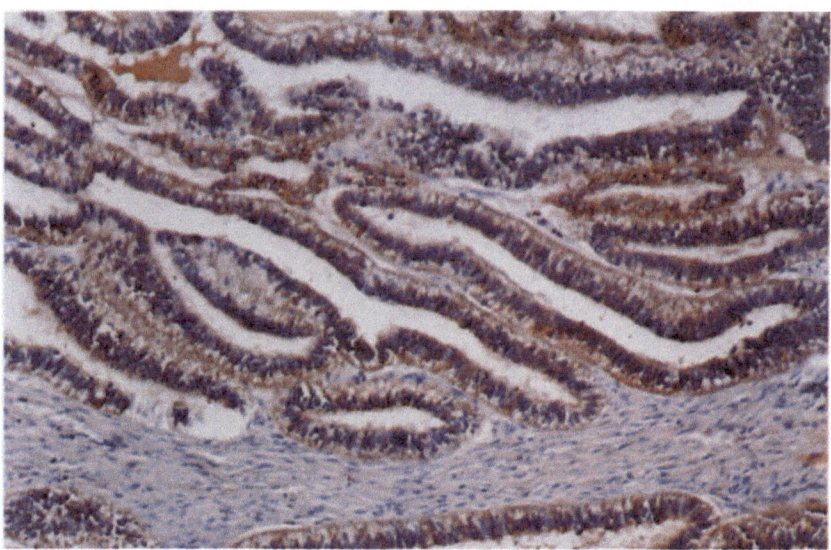

Fig. 102. *Glandular yolk sac tumacr.* Pattern resembling endometrioid adenocarcinoma but positive for a-fetoprotein. Immunoperoxidase stain

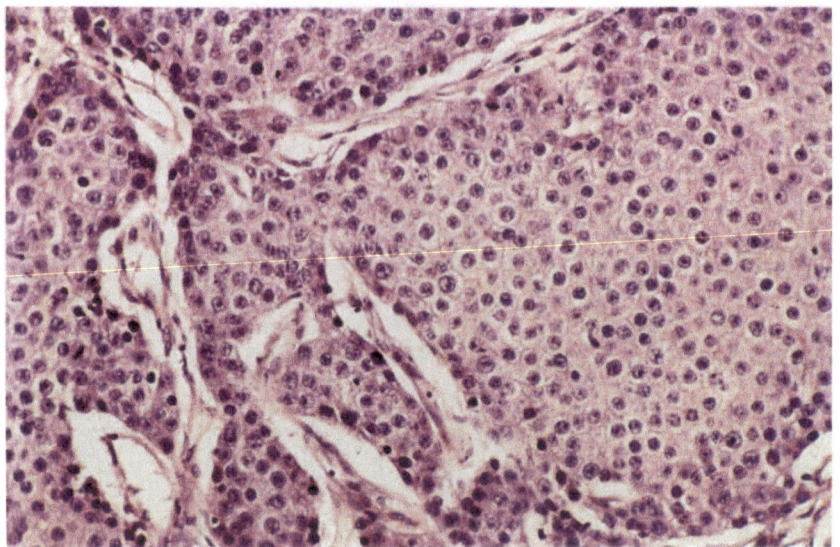

Fig. 103. *Hepatoid yolk sac tumour.* Resemblance to hepatocellular carcinoma

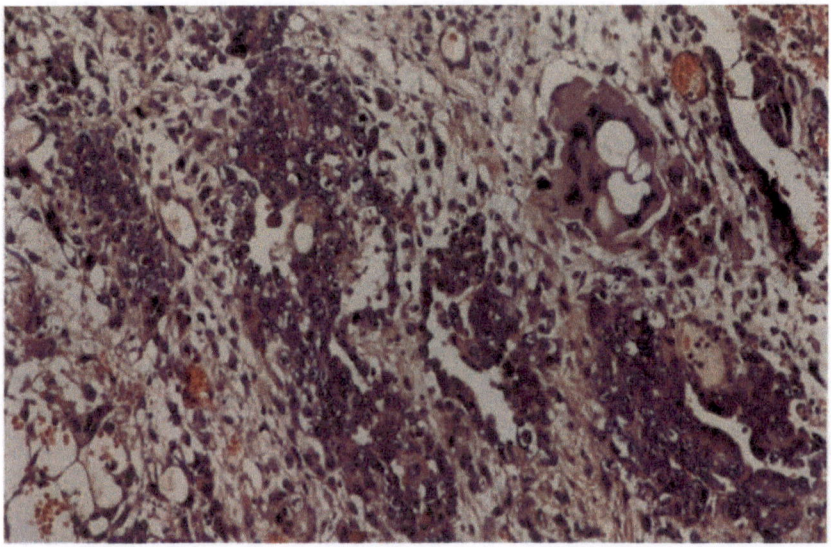

Fig. 104. *Embryonal carcinoma.* Groups of embryonal epithelial cells separated by cellular mesenchyme containing a syncytiotrophoblast cell

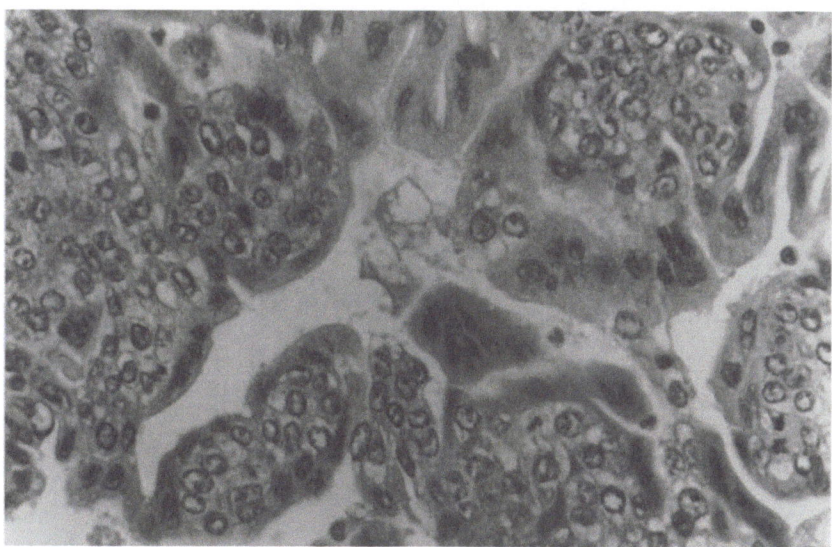

Fig. 105. *Choriocarcinoma.* Nodules of cytotrophoblast ringed by syncytiotrophoblast

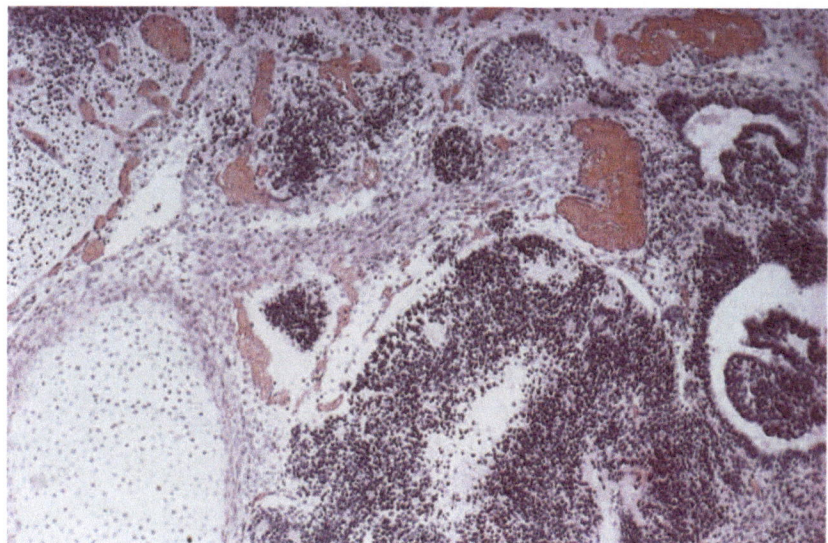

Fig. 106. *Immature teratoma.* Large nodule of primitive neuroectodermal cells with dark nuclei, cartilage and spaces lined by primitive epithelium

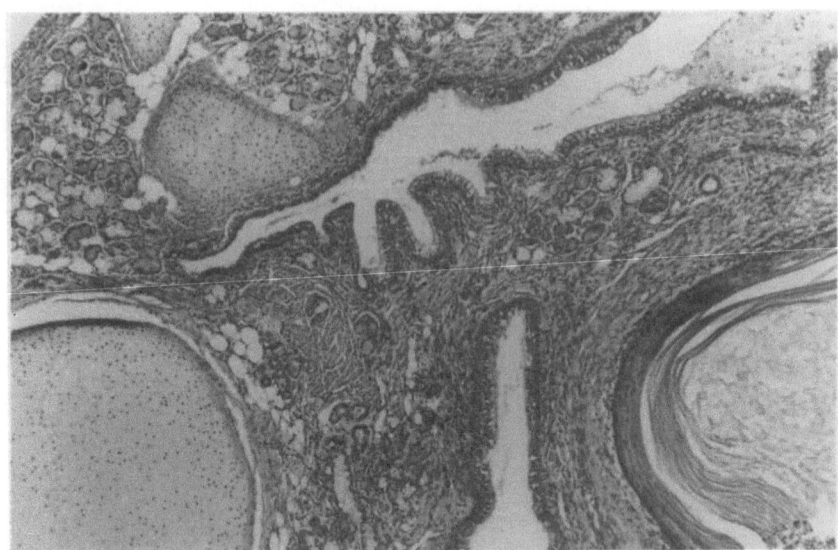

Fig. 107. *Mature teratoma, solid.* Nodules of cartilage and keratinizing squamous epithelium and elongated spaces lined by respiratory-type epithelium

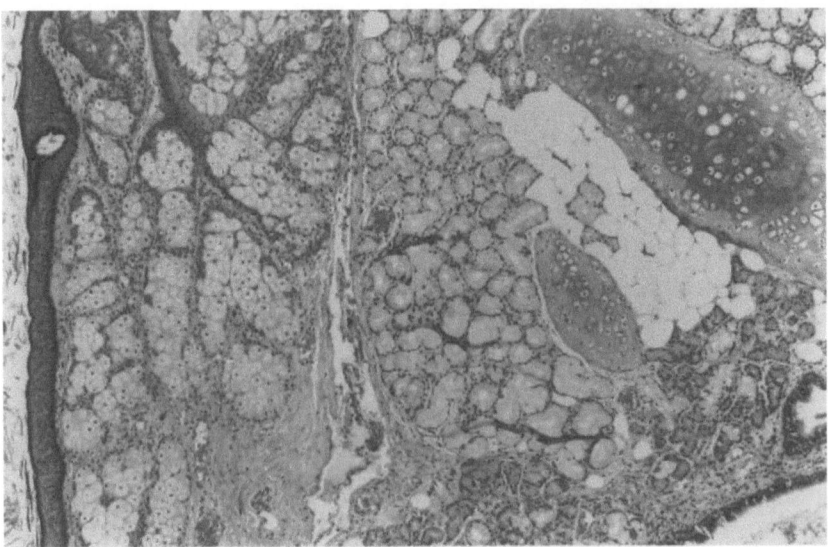

Fig. 108. *Mature cystic teratoma (dermoid cyst).* Cyst lined by squamous epithelium
with sebaceous glands and underlying salivary gland-type tissue, cartilage, fat and
space lined by respiratory epithelium *(lower right)*

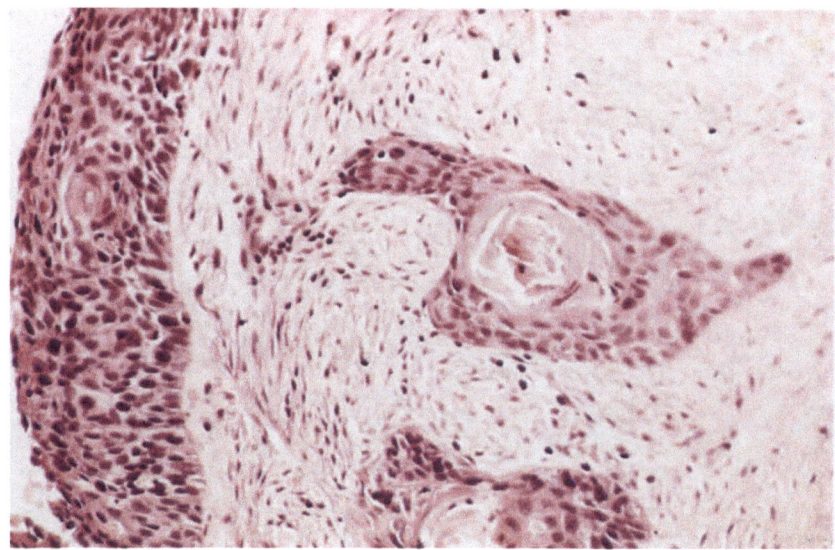

Fig. 109. *Mature cystic teratoma (dermoid cyst) with squamous cell carcinoma.* Invasive squamous cell nests underlying carcinoma in situ lining cyst. [From Scully RE, Young RH, Clement PB (1998) Tumors of the ovary, maldeveloped gonads, fallopian tube, and broad ligament. Atlas of tumor pathology, 3rd series. Armed Forces Institute of Pathology, Washington, DC]

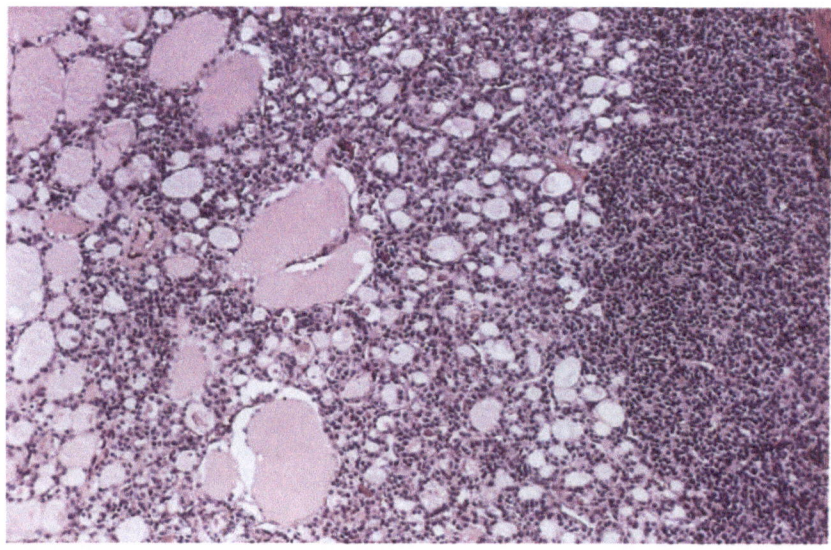

Fig. 110. *Struma ovarii with adenama.* Microfollicular, macrofollicular and embryonal patterns

110

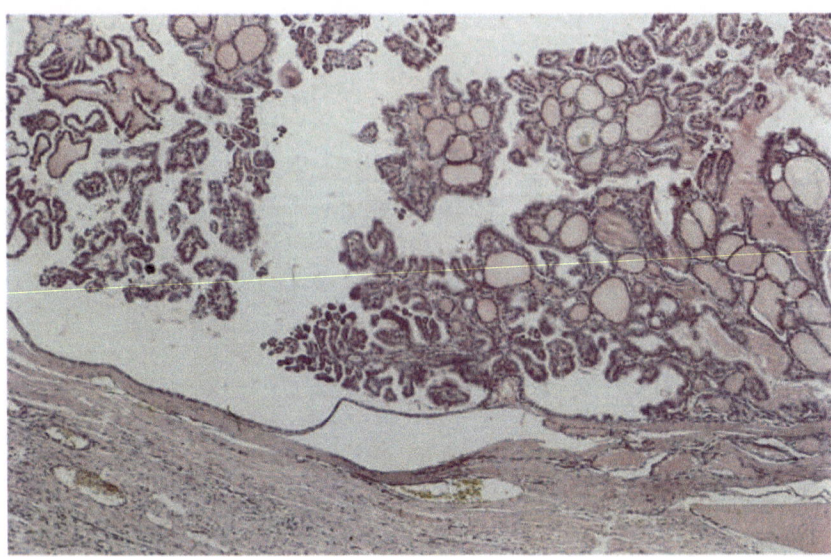

Fig. 111. *Struma ovarii with papillary carcinoma.* Papillary colloid-containing tumour protruding into lumen of cyst

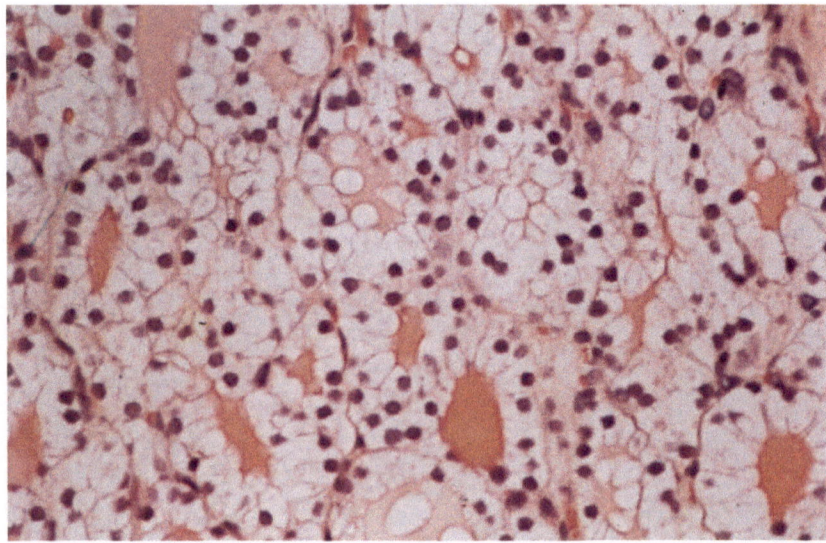

Fig. 112. *Struma ovarii with clear cell adenoma.* Clear cells enveloping collections of colloid. [From Scully RE, Young RH, Clement PB (1998) Tumors of the ovary, maldeveloped gonads, fallopian tube, and broad ligament. Atlas of tumor pathology, 3rd series. Armed Forces Institute of Pathology, Washington, DC]

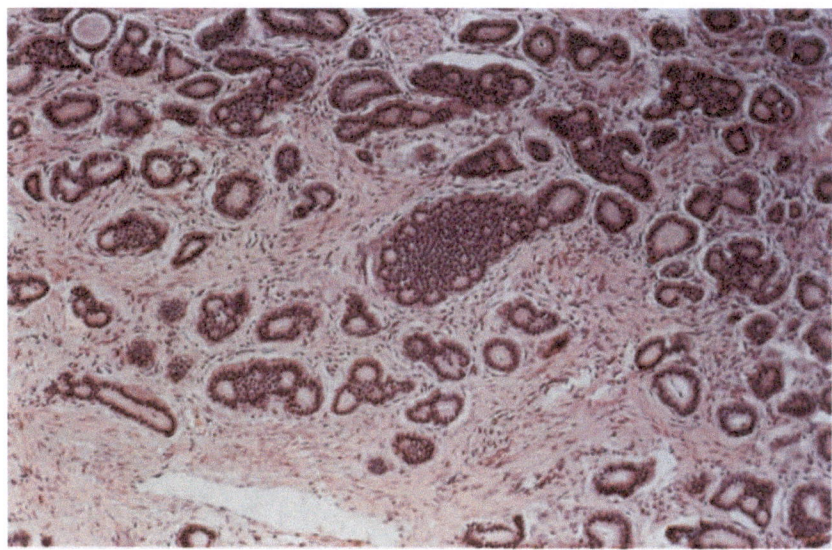

Fig. 113. *Carcinoid tumour, insular.* Rounded nests of cells with uniform dark nuclei and glands lined by similar cells lying in fibrous stroma. [From Young RH, Clement PB, Scully RE (1994) The ovary. In: Sternberg SS (ed) Diagnostic surgical pathology. Raven, New York, pp 2195–2279]

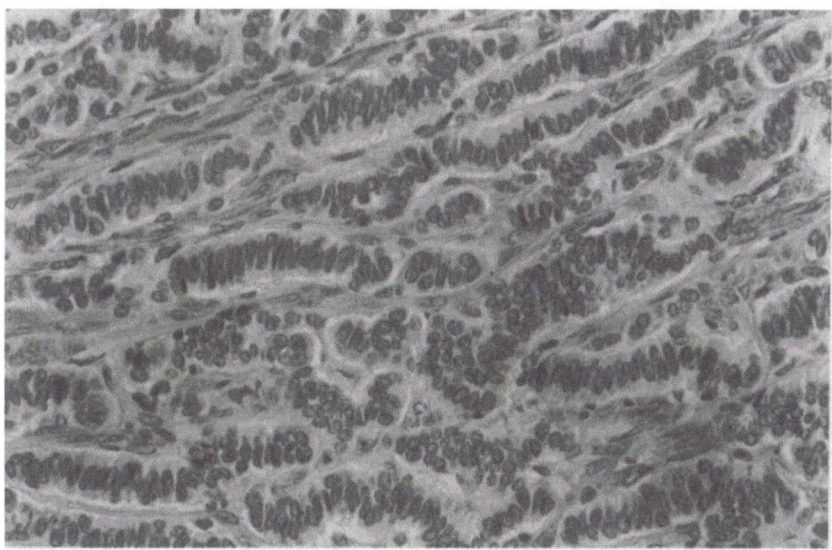

Fig. 114. *Carcinoid tumour, trabecular.* Ribbons of tumour cells separated by fibrous stroma

112

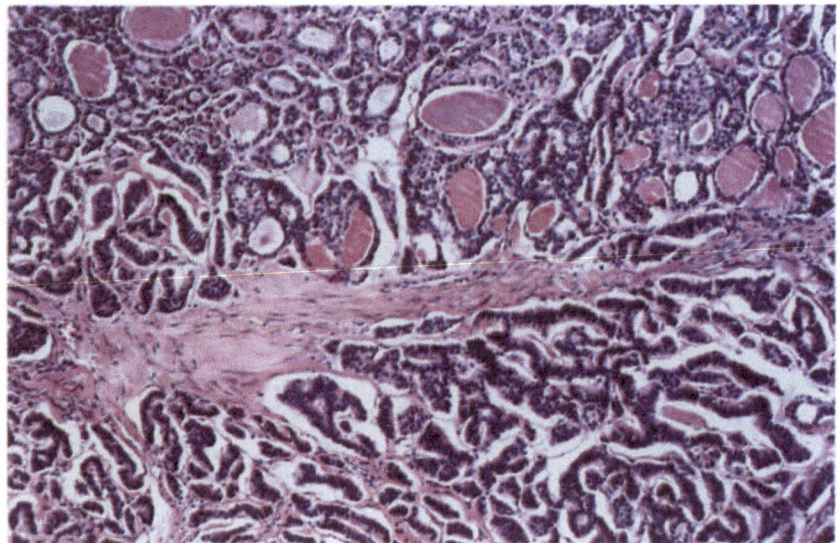

Fig. 115. *Strumal carcinoid tumour.* Ribbons of trabecular carcinoid tumour merging with follicles filled with colloid

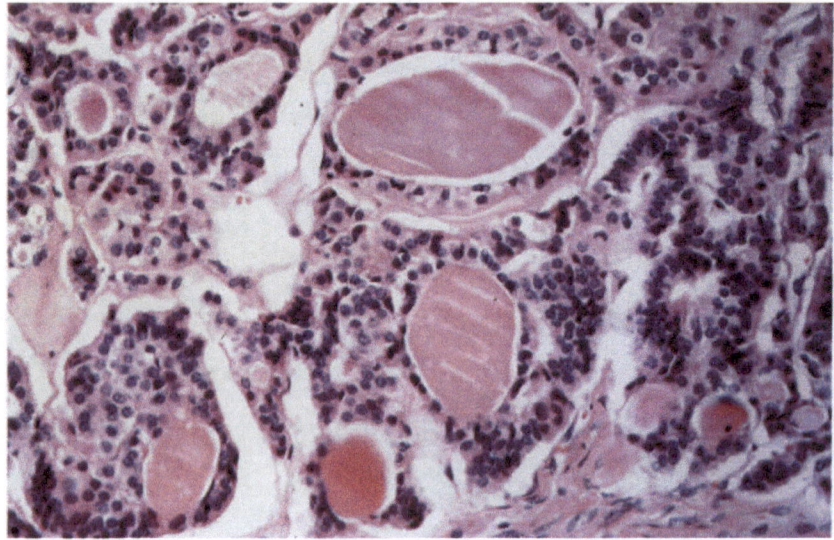

Fig. 116. *Strumal carcinoid tumour.* Carcinoid tumour cells surrounding colloid

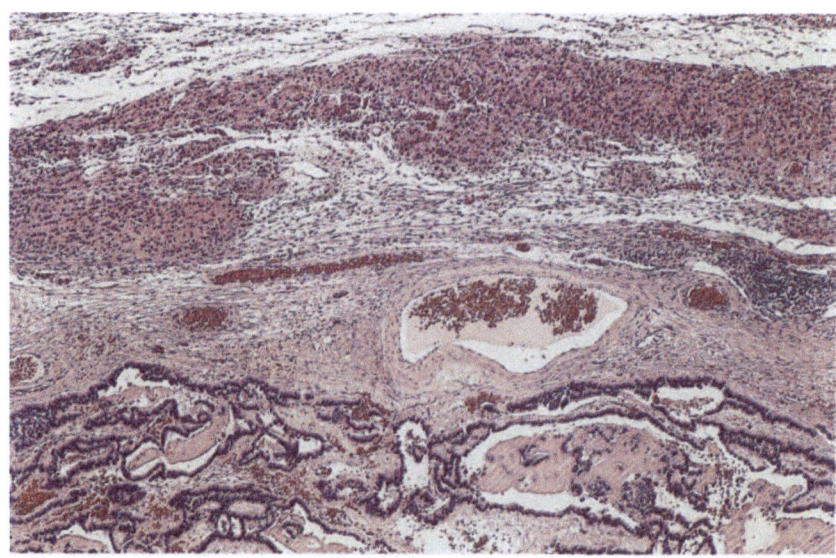

Fig. 117. *Strumal carcinoid tumour.* Peripheral band of steroid cells that contained crystals of Reinke adjacent to tumour. [From Scully RE, Young RH, Clement PB (1998) Tumors of the ovary, maldeveloped gonads, fallopian tube, and broad ligament. Atlas of tumor pathology, 3rd series. Armed Forces Institute of Pathology, Washington, DC]

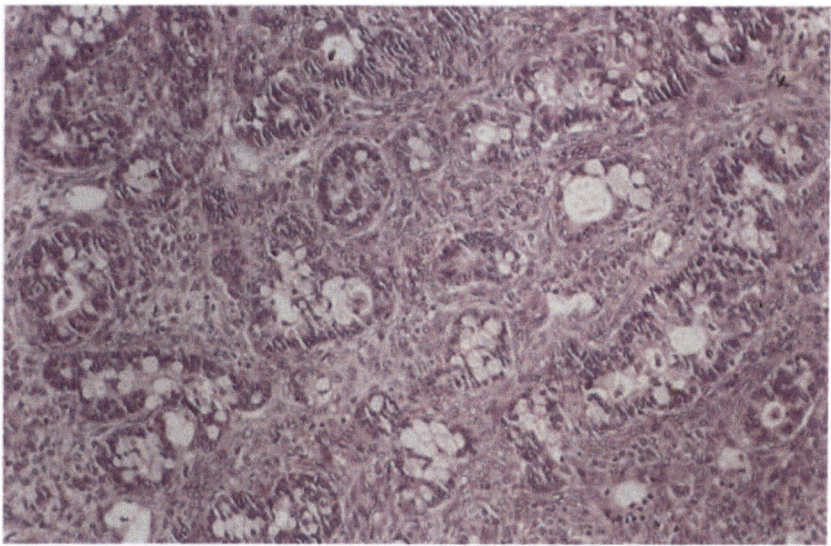

Fig. 118. *Goblet cell carcinoid tumour.* Nests and glands containing goblet cells lying in a cellular stroma. [From Scully RE, Young RH, Clement PB (1998) Tumors of the ovary, maldeveloped gonads, fallopian tube, and broad ligament. Atlas of tumor pathology, 3rd series. Armed Forces Institute of Pathology, Washington, DC]

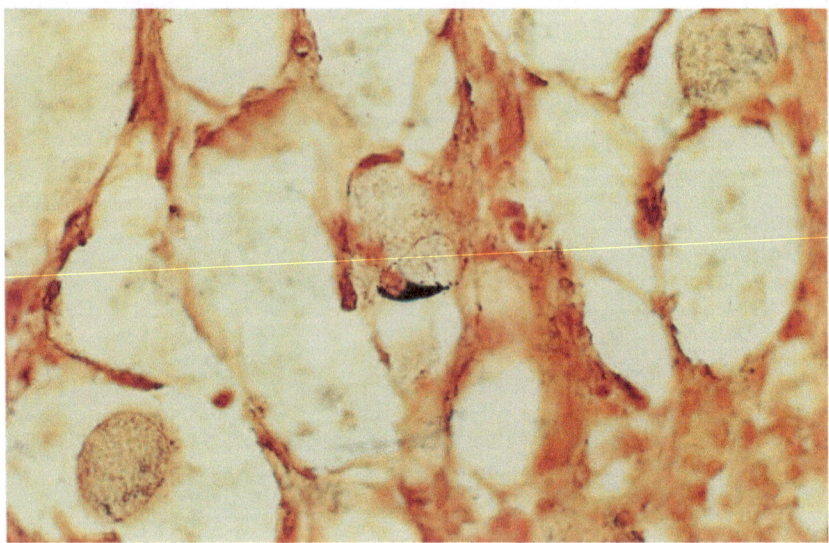

Fig. 119. *Goblet cell carcinoid tumour.* Goblet cell containing neuroendocrine granules *(center).* Grimelius stain

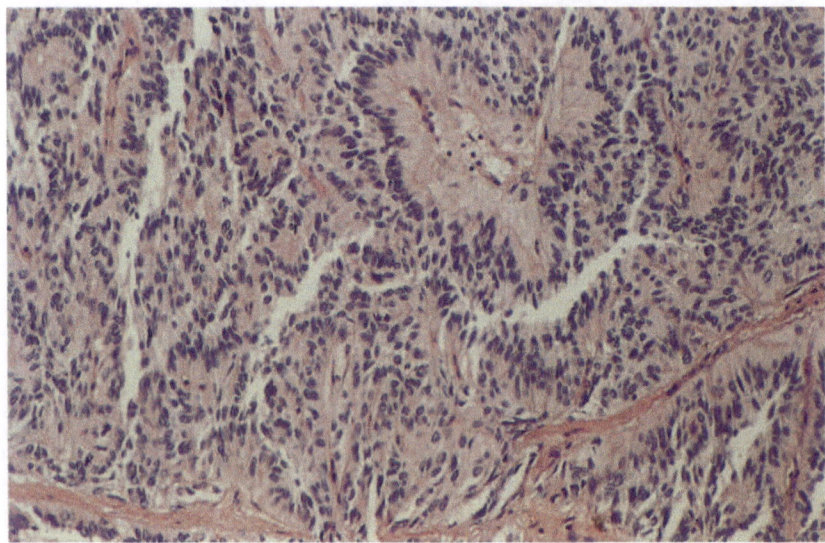

Fig. 120. *Ependymoma.* Pseudorosettes with apical nuclei of perivascular cells

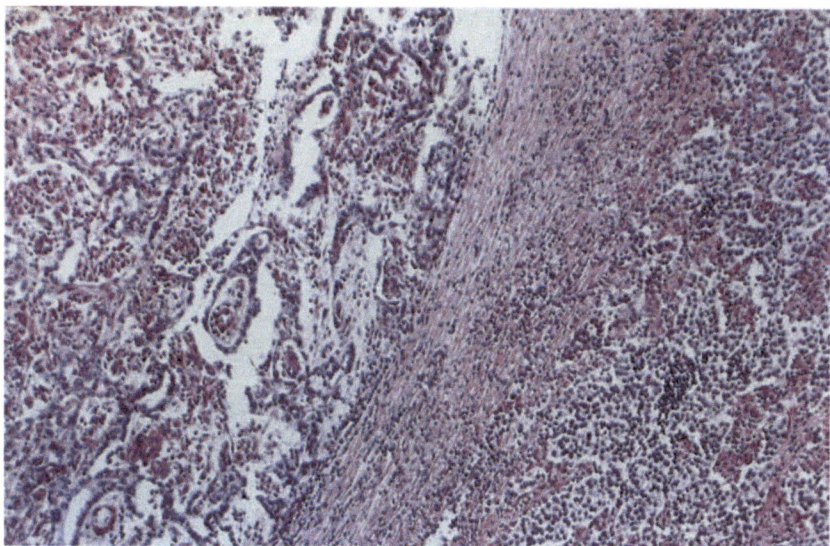

Fig. 121. *Mixed germ cell tumour.* Yolk sac tumour (*left*) and dysgerminoma (*right*). [From Scully RE, Young RH, Clement PB (1998) Tumors of the ovary, mal-developed gonads, fallopian tube, and broad ligament. Atlas of tumor pathology, 3rd series. Armed Forces Institute of Pathology, Washington, DC]

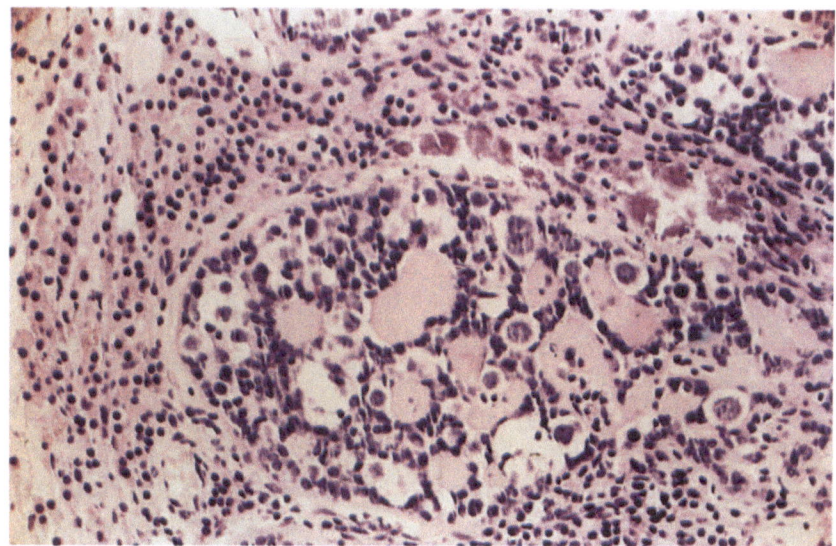

Fig. 122. *Gonadoblastoma.* Nest composed of germinoma-type cells and immature Sertoli cells surrounding hyaline nodules, adjacent to cells resembling Leydig cells

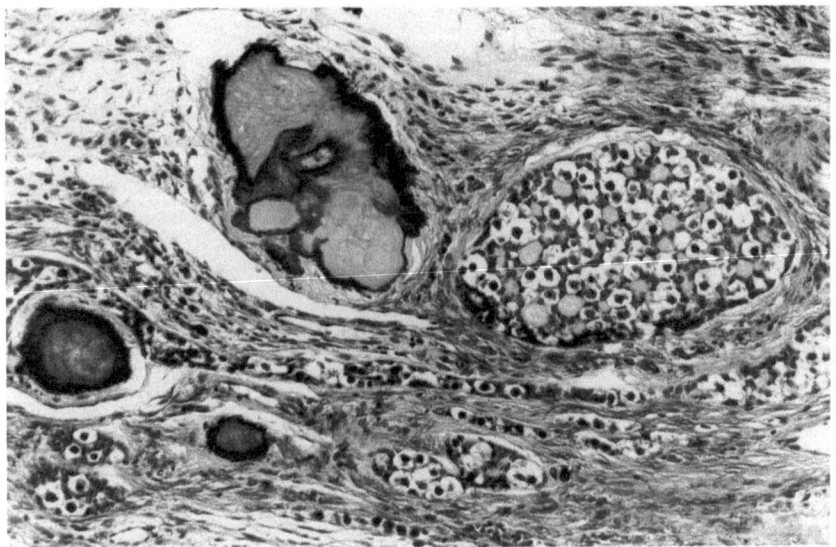

Fig. 123. *Gonadoblastoma.* Rounded foci of calcification

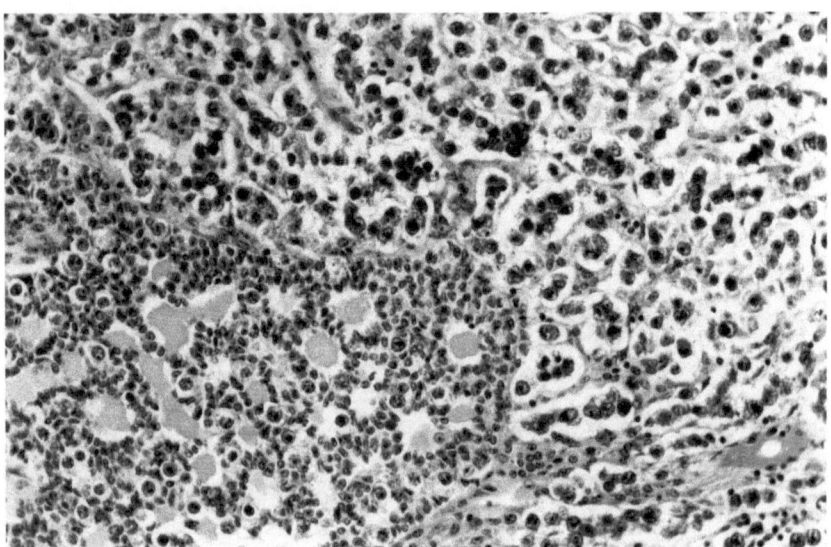

Fig. 124. *Gonadoblastoma with germinoma.* Germ cells infiltrating stroma

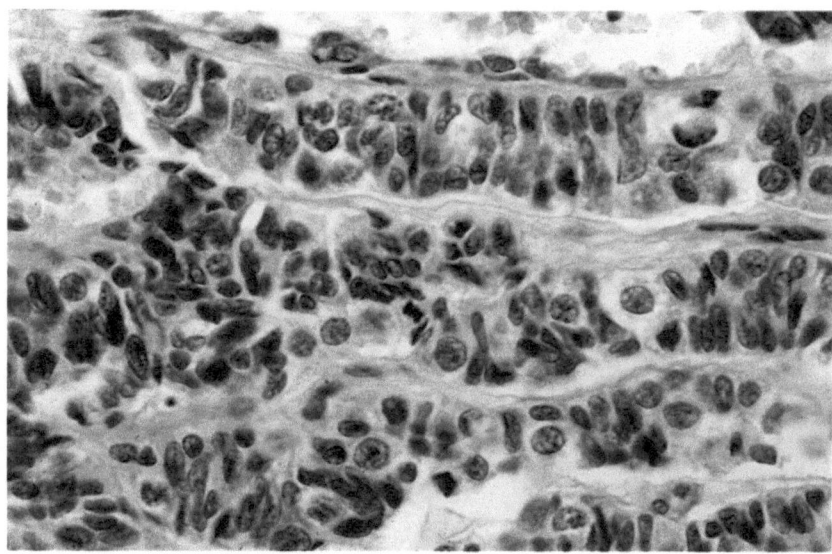

Fig. 125. *Germ cell-sex cord-stromal tumour of non-gonadoblastoma type.* Trabeculae composed of small cells of sex cord type with dark nuclei and scattered larger germ cells with large, round nuclei and abundant clear cytoplasm

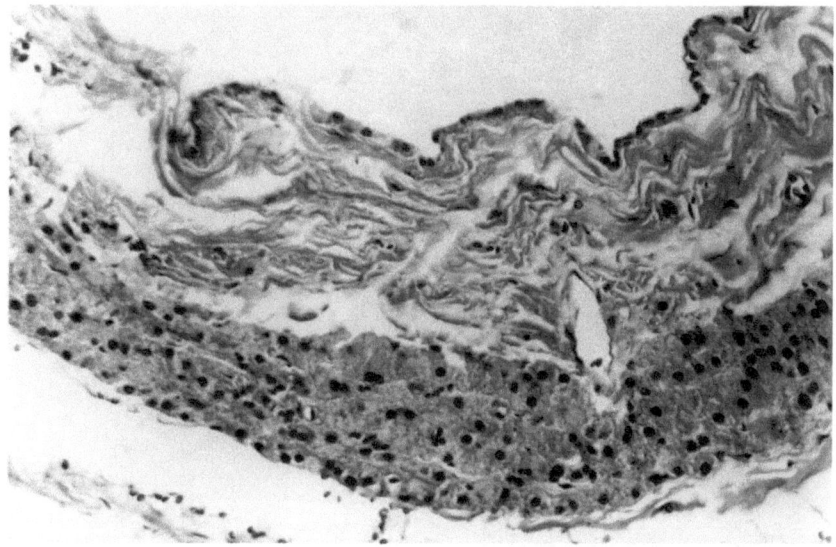

Fig. 126. *Rete cystadenoma.* Cyst lined by flat epithelium with crevices in its wall; adjacent band of hilar Leydig cells

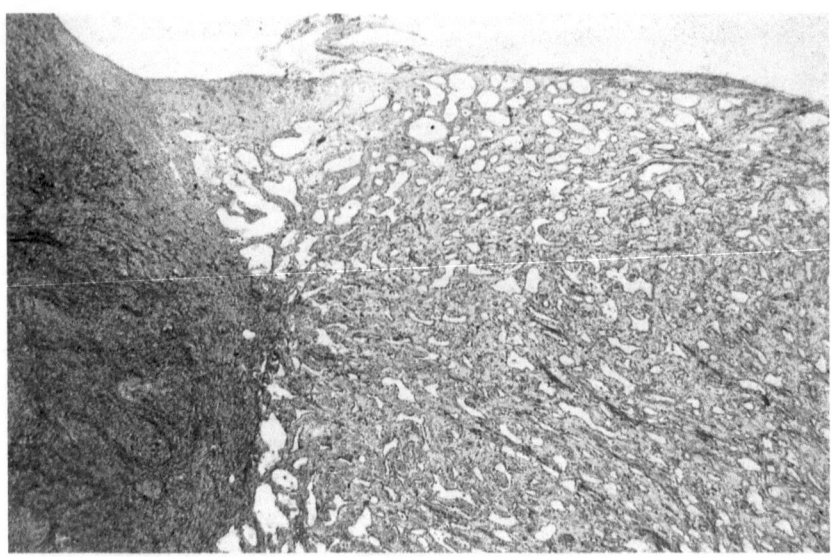

Fig. 127. *Adenomatoid tumour.* Tumour composed of small gland-like spaces and cysts lying in hilus. [From Scully RE, Young RH, Clement PB (1998) Tumors of the ovary, maldeveloped gonads, fallopian tube, and broad ligament. Atlas of tumor pathology, 3rd series. Armed Forces Institute of Pathology, Washington, DC]

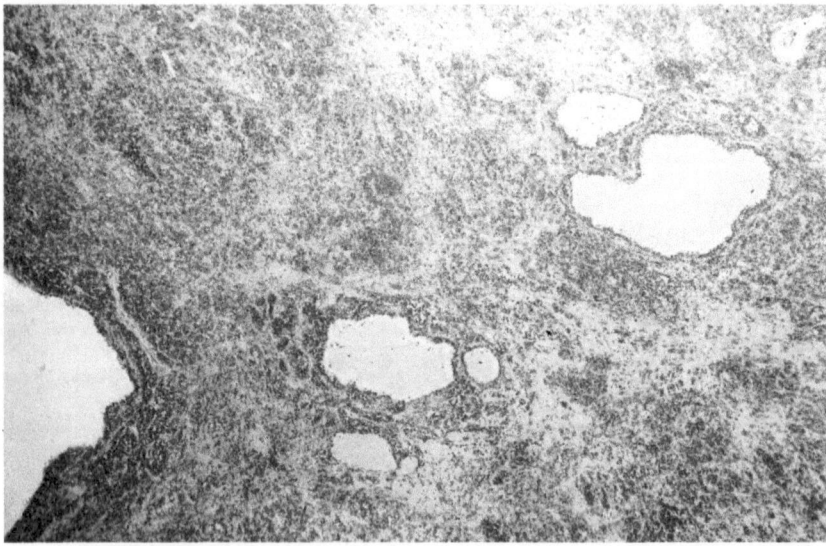

Fig. 128. *Small cell carcinoma, hypercalcaemic type.* Diffuse and nodular arrangement of small epithelial cells with follicle formation

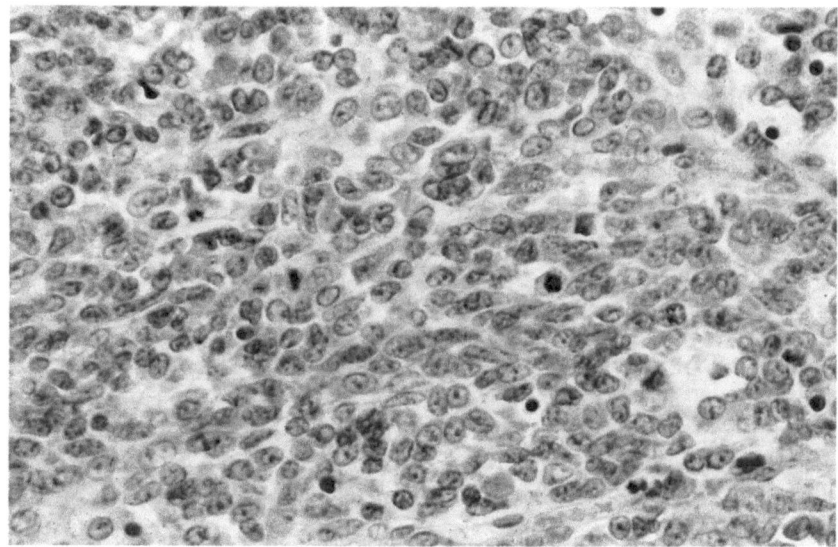

Fig. 129. *Small cell carcinoma, hypercalcaemic type.* Tumour cells with scanty cytoplasm and small round nuclei containing nucleoli and showing mitotic activity

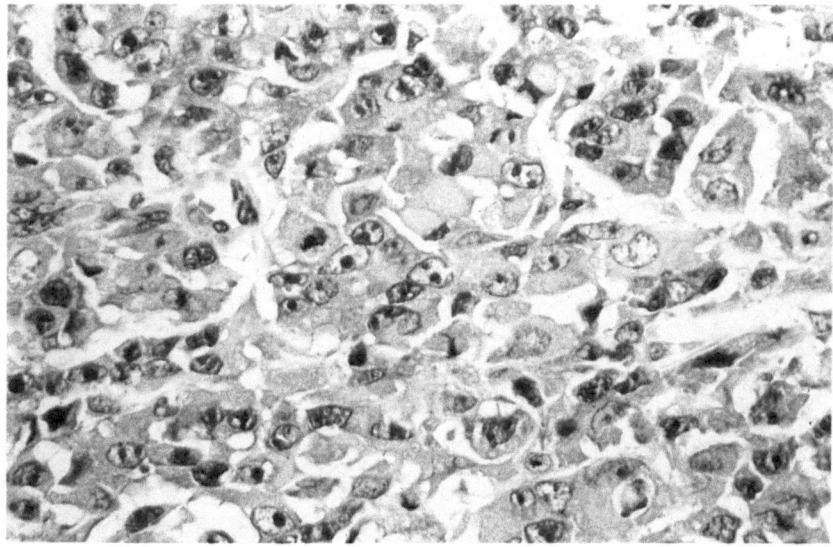

Fig. 130. *Small cell carcinoma, hypercalcaemic type.* Large cells with abundant eosinophilic cytoplasm and nuclei containing prominent nucleoli

120

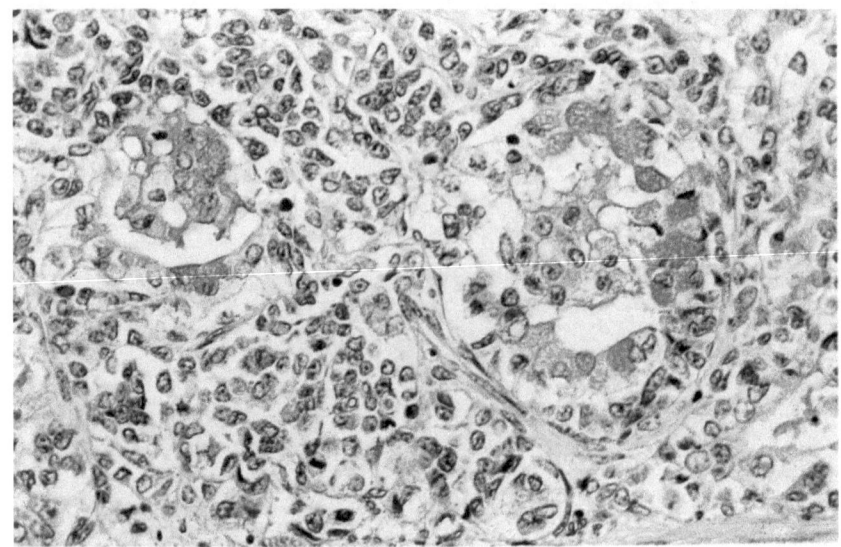

Fig. 131. *Small cell carcinoma, hypercalcaemic type*. Scattered tumour cells containing mucin. Mucicarmine stain

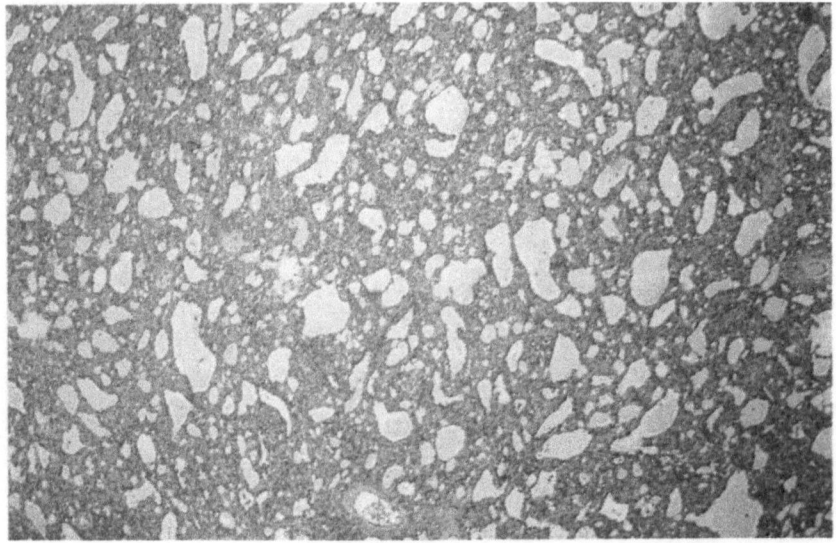

Fig. 132. *Tumour of probable wolffian origin*. Sieve-like pattern

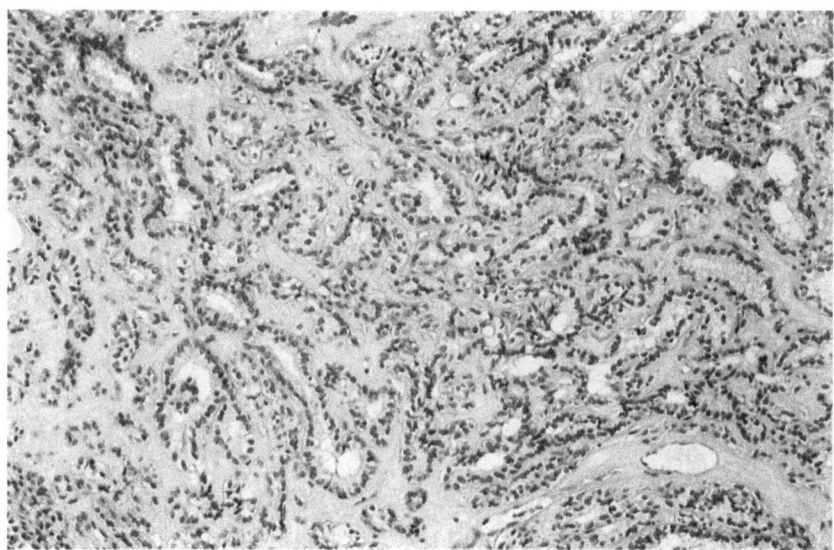

Fig. 133. *Tumour of probable wolffian origin.* Anastamosing tubules with lumens resembling those of Sertoli cell tumour. [From Scully RE, Young RH, Clement PB (1998) Tumors of the ovary, maldeveloped gonads, fallopian tube, and broad ligament. Atlas of tumor pathology, 3rd series. Armed Forces Institute of Pathology, Washington, DC]

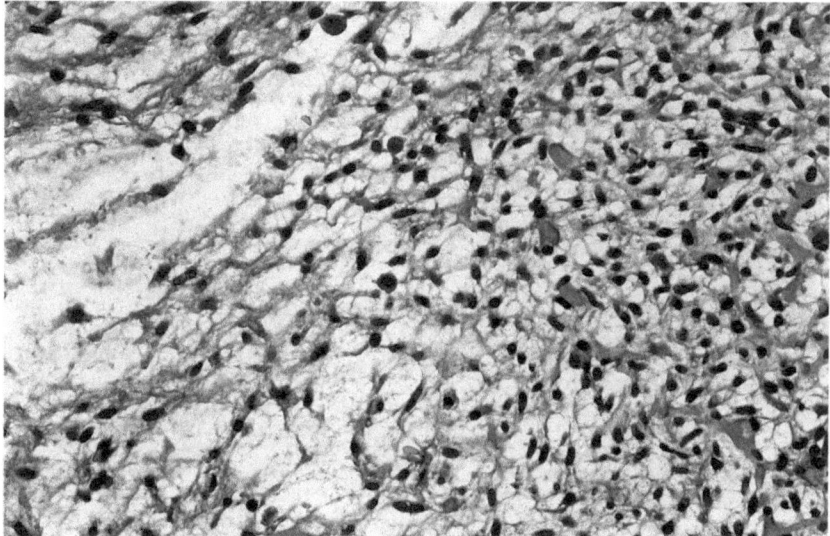

Fig. 134. *Myxoma.* Cells with spindle-shaped, oval and round nuclei separated by myxoid intercellular material

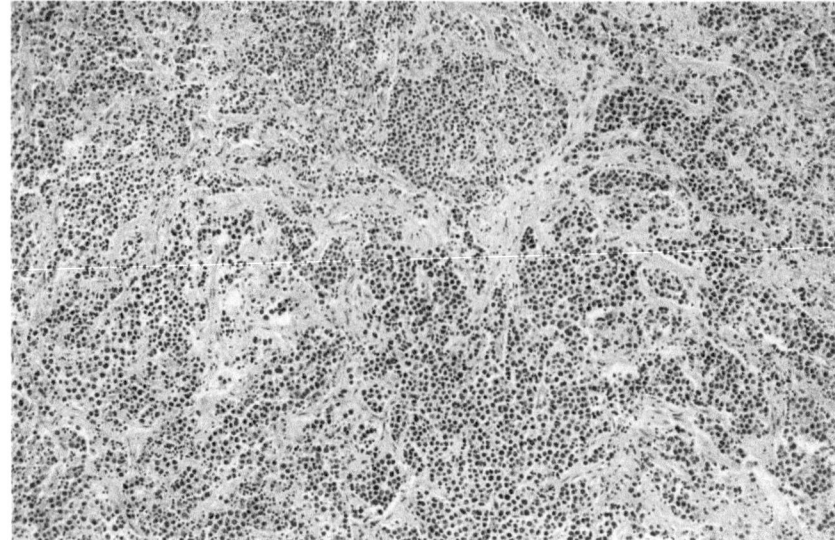

Fig. 135. *Lymphoma.* Nests and trabeculae of tumour cells separated by fibrous stroma, resembling pattern of carcinoma. [From Scully RE, Young RH, Clement PB (1998) Tumors of the ovary, maldeveloped gonads, fallopian tube, and broad ligament. Atlas of tumor pathology, 3rd series. Armed Forces Institute of Pathology, Washington, DC]

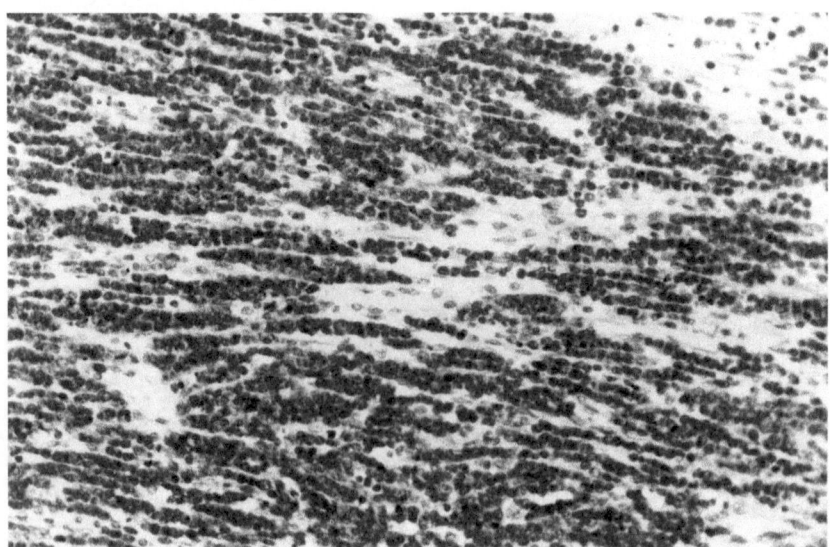

Fig. 136. *Lymphoma.* Growth in cords resembling pattern of carcinoma

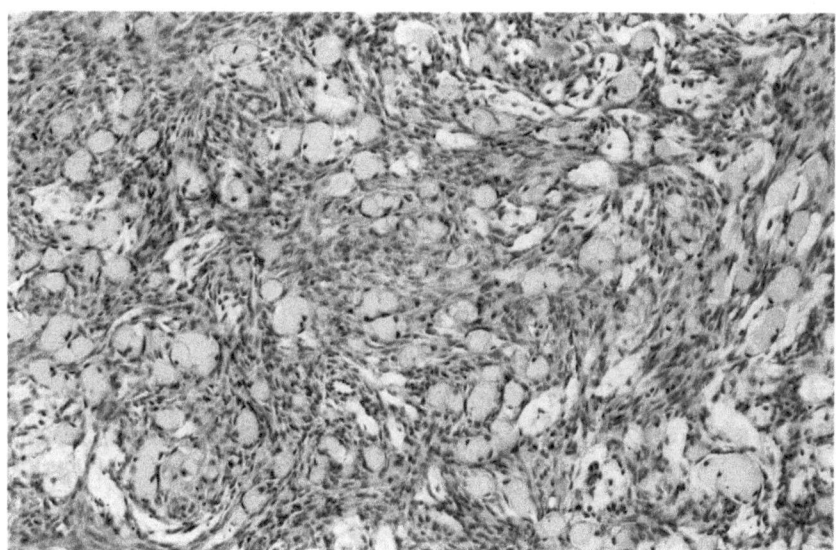

Fig. 137. *Krukenberg tumour.* Signet-ring cells in cellular stroma

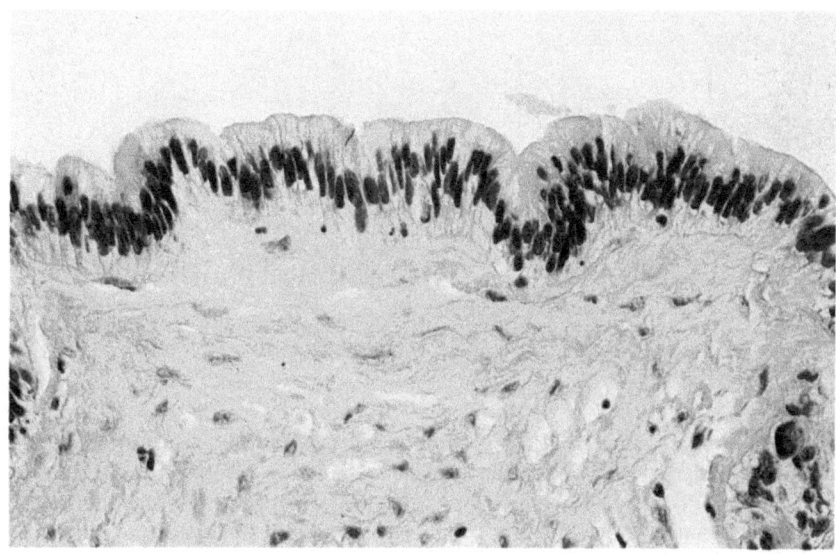

Fig. 138. *Metastatic adenocarcinoma from colon.* Cyst lined by benign-appearing epithelium

124

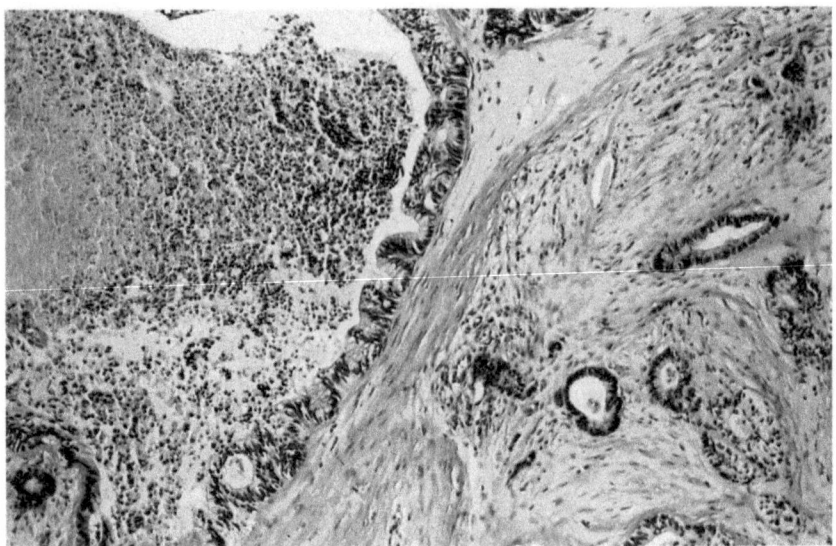

Fig. 139. *Metastatic adenocarcinoma from colon.* Cyst filled with "dirty" necrotic material adjacent to nodule composed of small glands in dense fibrous tissue

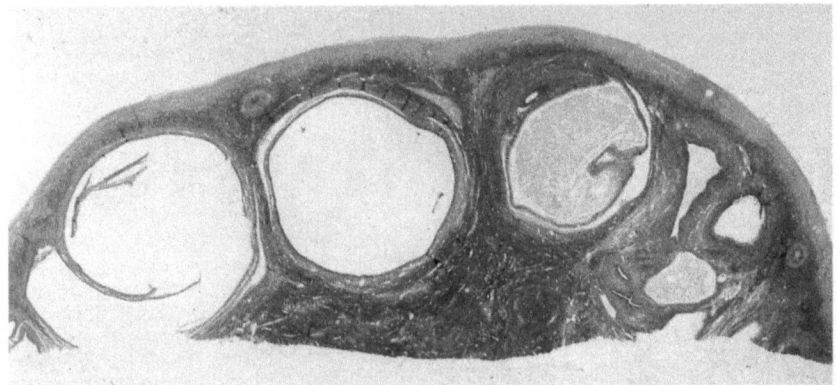

Fig. 140. *Multiple follicle cysts (polycystic ovarian disease).* Multiple follicle cysts in ovarian wedge specimen with collagenized outer cortex. [From Scully RE, Young RH, Clement PB (1998) Tumors of the ovary, maldeveloped gonads, fallopian tube, and broad ligament. Atlas of tumor pathology, 3rd series. Armed Forces Institute of Pathology, Washligton, DC]

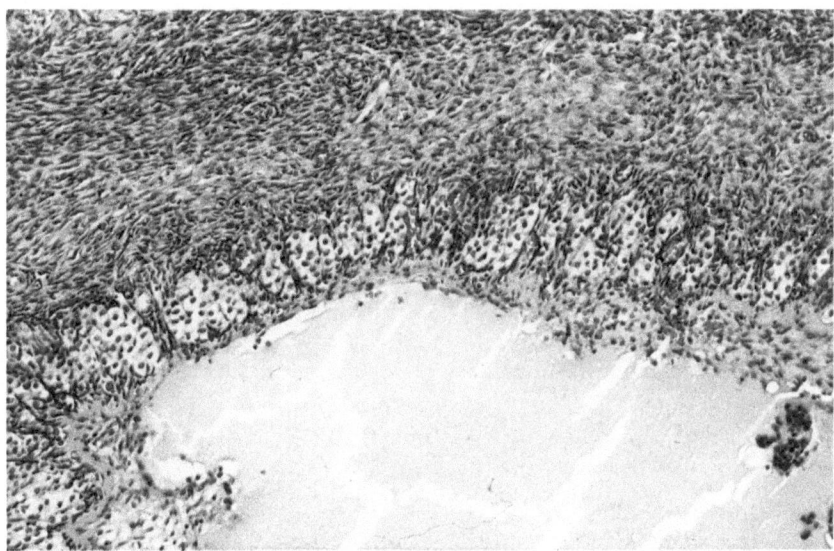

Fig. 141. *Multiple follicle cysts (polycystic ovarian disease).* Atretic follicle with thick layer of luteinized theca cells in wall. [From Scully RE, Young RH, Clement PB (1998) Tumors of the ovary, maldeveloped gonads, fallopian tube, and broad ligament. Atlas of tumor pathology, 3rd series. Armed Forces Institute of Pathology, Washington, DC]

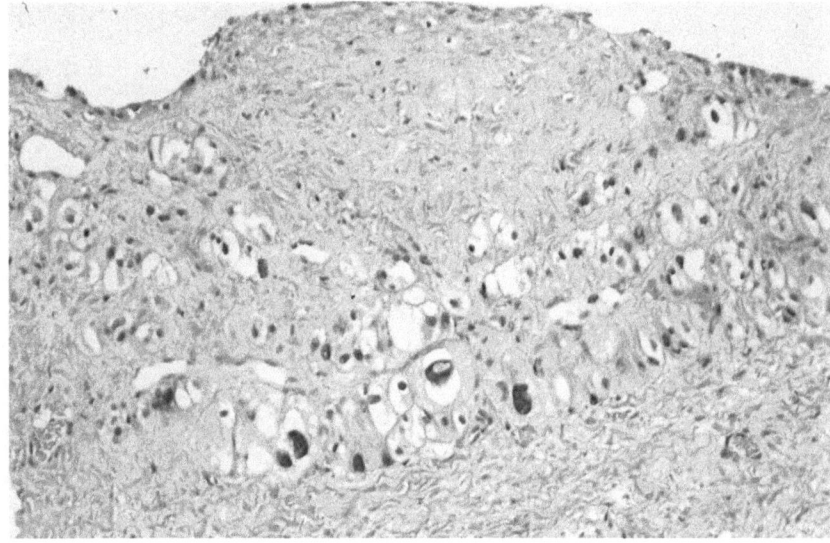

Fig. 142. *Large solitary luteinized follicle cyst of pregnancy and puerperium.* Bizarre nuclei in luteinized cells in cyst wall

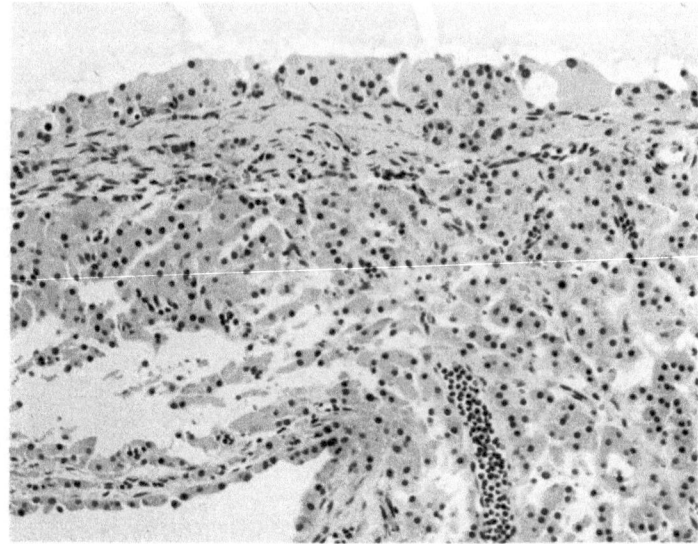

Fig. 143. *Hyperreactio luteinalis.* Luteinization of granulosa cell and particularly theca cell layers of follicles. [From Scully RE, Young RH, Clement PB (1998) Tumors of the ovary, maldeveloped gonads, fallopian tube, and broad ligament. Atlas of tumor pathology, 3rd series. Armed Forces Institute of Pathology, Washington, DC]

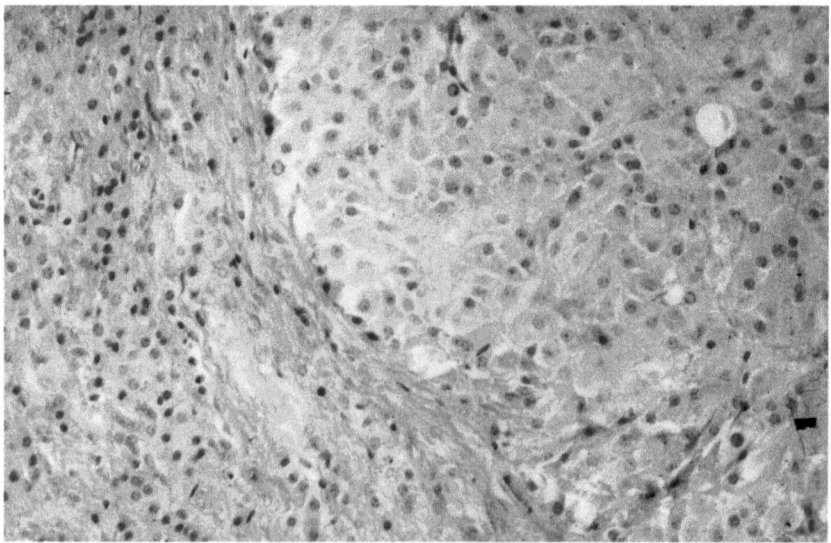

Fig. 144. *Pregnancy luteoma.* Luteoma (*right*) adjacent to luteinized theca cells (*left*) in wall of follicle (not seen)

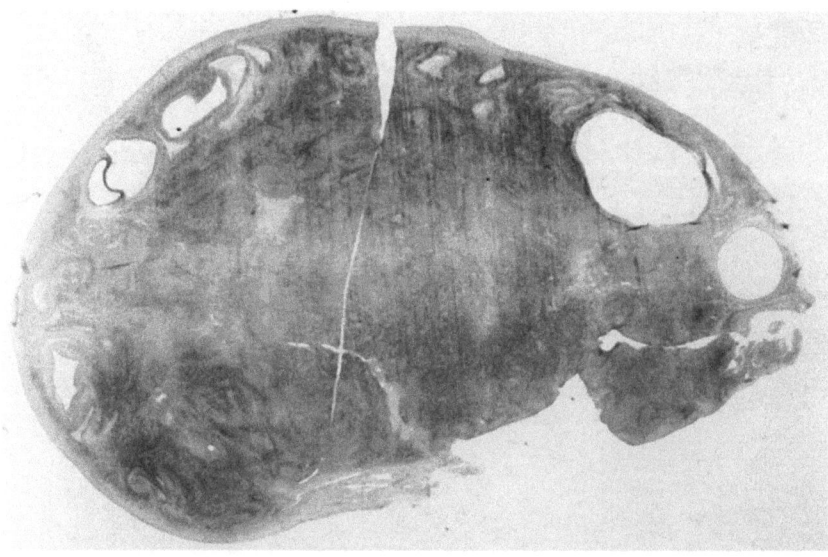

Fig. 145. *Stromal hyperthecosis.* Most of ovary replaced by hyperplastic stroma with residual peripheral follicle cysts and collagenization of outer cortex

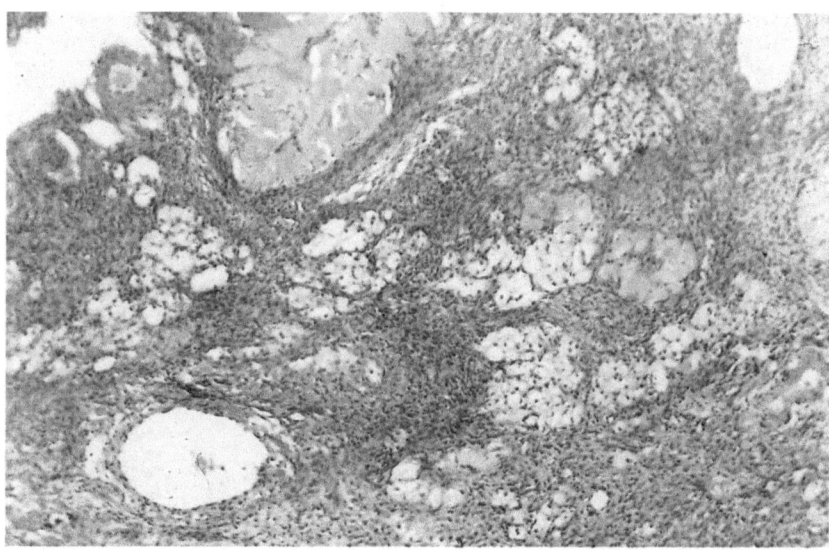

Fig. 146. *Stromal hyperthecosis.* Nests of luteinized lipid-rich stromal cells in hyperplastic stroma

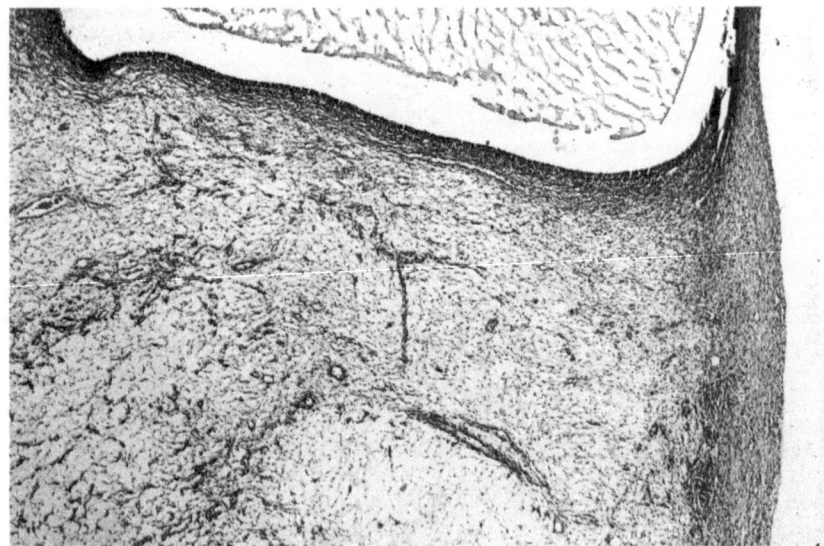

Fig. 147. *Massive oedema.* Markedly oedematous ovarian stroma enclosing cystic follicle with collagenization of outer cortex

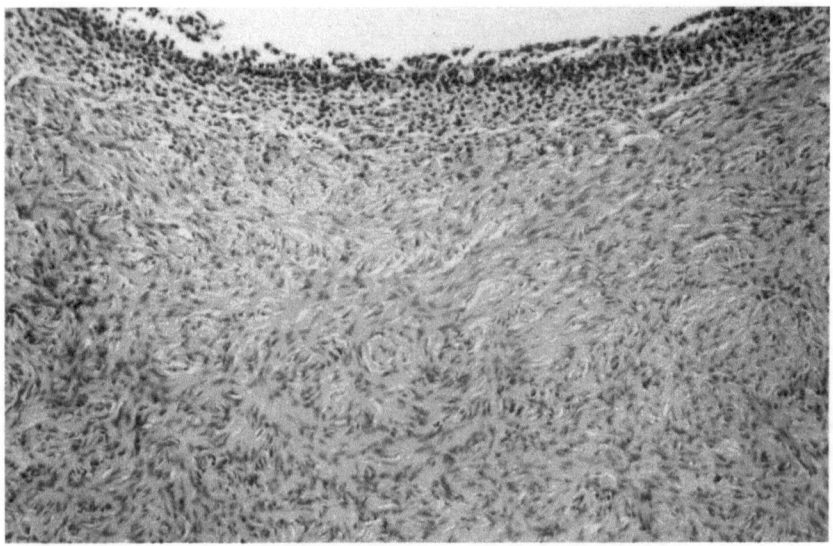

Fig. 148. *Fibromatosis.* Fibromatous tissue enveloping graafian follicle

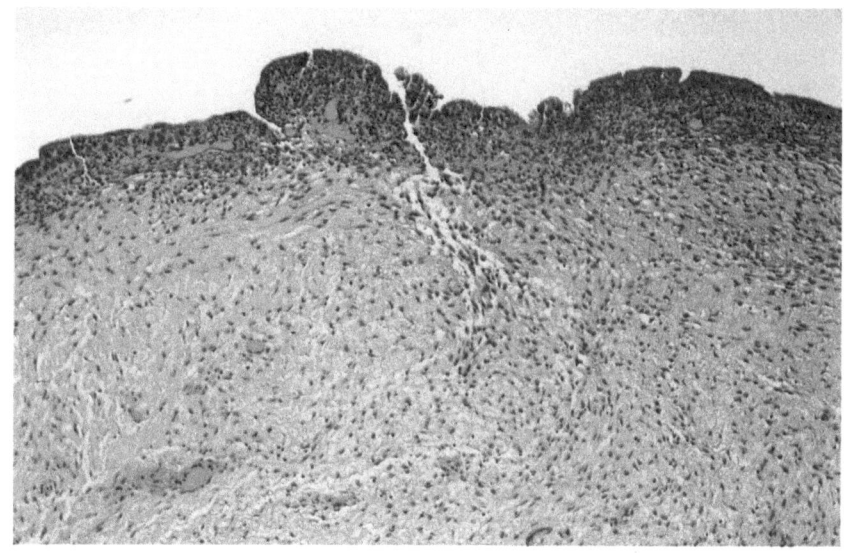

Fig. 149. *Endometriosis.* Endometriotic cyst with predominant component of dense fibrous tissue

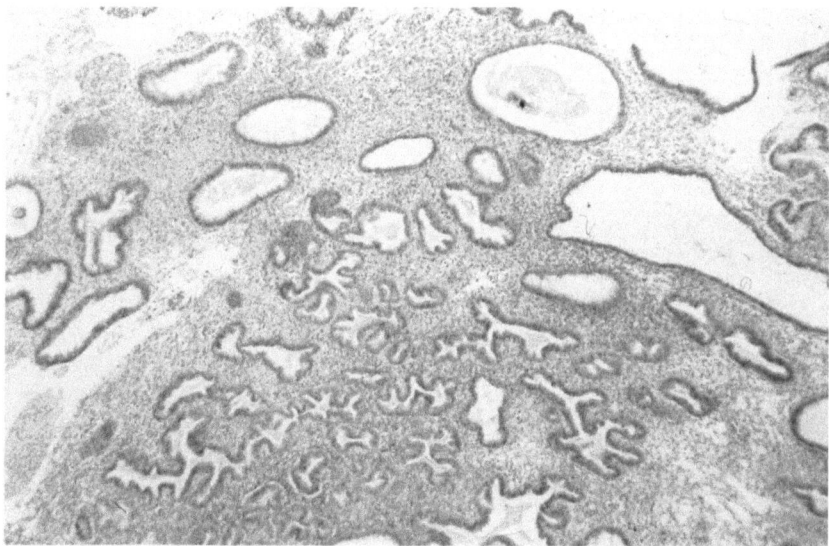

Fig. 150. *Endometriosis.* Simple and complex hyperplasia

Subject Index